T0296062

THE
ENDEAVOUR OF JEAN FERNEL

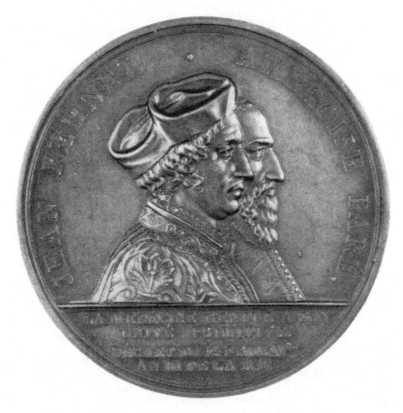

Obverse of the Fernel-Paré Medal, struck in the eighteenth century.
[Fig. 11.]

THE ENDEAVOUR OF JEAN FERNEL

WITH A

List of the Editions of his Writings

BY

SIR CHARLES SHERRINGTON, O.M.

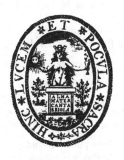

CAMBRIDGE
AT THE UNIVERSITY PRESS
1946

To

E. N. da C. ANDRADE, F.R.S.
gratefully for his interest
in this brief study

CAMBRIDGE
UNIVERSITY PRESS

University Printing House, Cambridge CB2 8BS, United Kingdom

Cambridge University Press is part of the University of Cambridge.

It furthers the University's mission by disseminating knowledge in the pursuit of
education, learning and research at the highest international levels of excellence.

www.cambridge.org
Information on this title: www.cambridge.org/9781107453784

© Cambridge University Press 1946

First published 1946
First paperback edition 2014

A catalogue record for this publication is available from the British Library

ISBN 978-1-107-45378-4 Paperback

Cambridge University Press has no responsibility for the persistence or accuracy of
URLs for external or third-party internet websites referred to in this publication,
and does not guarantee that any content on such websites is, or will remain, accurate
or appropriate.

Contents

I. Biographical notices of Fernel: Guillaume Plancy. II. Plancy's 'Life' of Fernel. III. Clichtoveus. IV. 'Insidiosæ Pacis'. V. Jacques Govea. VI. Goulin's researches regarding Fernel. VII. Shellfish and the moon. VIII. Valcher's tractates. IX. Riolan the Elder's works on Fernel. X. The fatal tourney-wound of Henri II of France. XI. Other portraits of Fernel. XII. Guy Patin. XIII. The text of the 'Physiology' of 1554. XIV. Boerhaave's recommendation of books for medical curriculum. XV. Nicolas Leonicenus. XVI. Thomas Linacre. XVII. Passage in the Pathologia, 1567. XVIII. Laurent Joubert's Paradoxes. XIX. Fracastor on cause of syphilis.

Illustrations

The Endpapers show a plan of part of old Paris simplified from Ph. Renouard.

Preface

Prefacing this small volume let me thank those who in one way or another have helped its preparation: Professor E. N. da C. Andrade, Mr Angus and Professor Dean, Master of Trinity Hall, Professor D. Denny-Brown of Harvard University, Professor Munro Fox, F.R.S., Dr John Fulton, Sterling Professor at Yale, Mr E. P. Goldsmidt, Professor Laignel-Lavastine of Paris, Professor Gilbert Murray, Professor F. M. Powicke, Dr V. Scholderer of the British Museum, Professor A. Souter, F.B.A., and not least, Regius Professor W. W. Buckland, Mr Henry Deas, and Mr Eric Blackall, of this College. Professor Andrade has read the text through and given me his comments. In the appended list of editions of Fernel I have had the advantage of consultation with Professor John Fulton and with Dr H. M. Sinclair, bibliographers whose shelves are especially rich in editions of Fernel. I have further consulted a number of librarians whom I would here thank; among them Mr H. M. Adams, Trinity College Library, Cambridge, Mr Thomas Graham, Royal College of Physicians' Library, Edinburgh, Mr Philip Grierson, Librarian of Gonville and Caius College, the Librarian of the Hunterian Collection, University of Glasgow, Mr G. F. Home, Royal Society of Medicine, London, Mr Le Fanu, Royal College of Surgeons of England, Mr H. W. Robinson of the Royal Society Library, Mr Scholfield and his staff of the University Library, Cambridge, Dr W. D. Simpson, University of Aberdeen, Dr H. Thomas, F.B.A., Keeper of Printed Books in the British Museum.

The book had its origin in a Thomas Vicary Lecture I was privileged to give at the Royal College of Surgeons, London. The theme is an old-time reform of Medicine, outstanding in its own sixteenth century, though not one of those commanding developments of knowledge such as were to transform Medicine and Surgery in a later age. Its author was perhaps the most learned and considered physician of his century, but he condemned the self-complacency of the orthodox Medicine of the time, and its belief that the Golden Age of Medicine had at last arrived. Not so he. He repudiated two systems of learning which, appealing to magic and the occult, eked out and smoothed over the failures and misadventures of Medicine. He taught that the best assured ground of Medicine is the universality of 'natural law'. In that he was a reformer, and is a factor in the creation of our Medicine of to-day.

C. S. S.

GONVILLE AND CAIUS COLLEGE
CAMBRIDGE
1945

Part I

THE STRUGGLE & ITS AIMS

I SUPPOSE that, for our purpose, Galen 'On the Use of the Parts' (περὶ χρείας μορίων) may be taken to be the earliest separate treatise dealing with human physiology. For more than thirteen centuries it found no successor. The attempt to fill such a gap must have required both a conviction and a certain courage. The man who ventured was Jean Fernel. He called his book 'The Natural Part of Medicine', and issued it in Paris in the year 1542. He was already eminent as a physician, and greatly occupied in practice and in teaching. The book was, as was Galen's, a physiology contributory to medicine. It had an immediate vogue. It met a need. Fernel had judged rightly in thinking there was room for it. His treatise was issued again and again, in Venice and Lyons as well as in Paris. He changed its name to 'Physiology'. For more than a century it remained *the* treatise on its subject. Harvey's discovery of the circulation of the blood in the following century, on becoming generally accepted, at last put Fernel's treatise out of date. But the compendious name, 'physiology', which he had given to the subject, has continued in use ever since.

Who was Jean Fernel? His publishers styled him 'philosopher and physician'. His early years ran briefly thus. Son of a substantial furrier and innkeeper at Montdidier, he was twelve years old when his parents moved to Clermont in Beauvoisis, twenty miles from Paris. Fernel as an author called himself 'of Amiens', *Ambianus*, perhaps because his father's family was originally from Amiens, perhaps because Montdidier was in the diocese of Amiens. But he got his schooling at Clermont, and seems to have shown early an ambition to go on to the University, at Paris. His parents yielded to that wish, though tardily.[1] At the University, the Collège de Ste Barbe, of old and good repute,[2] received him. He followed the

---

[1] Plancy—and on him we have to rely for most of this part of Fernel's story—is at pains to say that to the paternal sympathy, not the maternal, the lad owed the indulgence of being sent to Paris for a university career.

[2] Founded in 1460, as an offshoot from the great Collège de Navarre.

course for M.A. Goulin thinks he was probably excused grammar as having already learnt it well at school. The headship of the Collège de Ste Barbe during the second and third decades of the fifteenth century was distinguished and progressive. It was held by the Goveas, Jacques and then his nephew André. Montaigne, who came under André Govea later at Bordeaux, said of him that he was 'the best teacher in all France'.

Fernel did well at College. On taking the M.A. degree he was invited more than once to stay on and teach dialectics. He was then twenty-two only; but Jean Jacques de Mesmes was lecturing publicly on law at Toulouse before he was twenty, and Louis de Bourges is said to have lectured publicly on medicine in Paris when he was twenty-three. Fernel declined the offers. Guillaume Plancy,[1] for ten years Fernel's assistant and living in his house, wrote on his master's death, a short 'Life' which is the chief biography.[2] He enters at some length into Fernel's academic outlook and situation at the time of the taking of his degree. Plancy held it to have been a critical juncture in his master's whole career. He says, Fernel 'desired by private study to acquaint himself better with the writings of Cicero, Aristotle and Plato'. What he would hitherto have had in his hands would have been compendia—'Expositiones' and 'Flores', containing essentials, chiefly in view of disputation for examination. One such was the Flores of Peter Mercarius, a physics and cosmology condensed from Aristotle and Ptolemy, published in Paris, in 1517 (1516 O.S.). In Goulin's chronology of Fernel, this would be two years before his taking his M.A. It was issued and sold by Oliver Senant, at the 'sign of Ste Barbe', half-way down the rue St Jacques, just below the Church of St Benoît. It is a folio, of twenty-six leaves, containing sets of numbered propositions, each proposition followed by an 'answer' called a 'correlation'. Mercarius, its author, was, at the time, a tutor at the 'famous' (*praeclarissimum*) Collège de Coqueret. He dedicates it, in sprightly terms of affection, to five *conphilosophantes*, among them John de Celaya, eminent Thomist, a 'Vicar General'. The Collège de Coqueret was one of the sixty-eight Parisian Colleges founded before 1500.[3] It was a little younger than Fernel's own Ste Barbe, and situate next door but one to it. It was in Fernel's

---

1 Note I, *v. infra, Appendix*, p. 147.
2 An extenso translation of it is given in Note II, *Appendix*, p. 150.
3 Geoffroi Tory, the painter and engraver, taught there, 1506.

lifetime to be a nurse of that literary child of the French Renaissance, the Pléiade; in 1549 Ronsard produced there his french version of Aristophanes' *Plutus*.

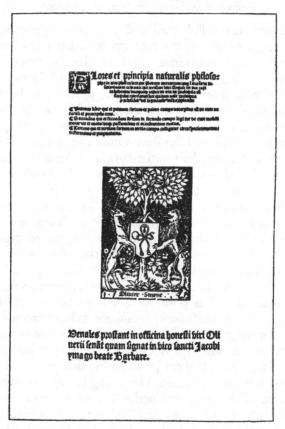

Fig. 1. Mercarius' *Flores*, 2°. Senant was printing 1505-25. An emblem of his bears:

En ce monde fault bien tirer
Qui en Paradis Veult monter.

Fernel's intention 'by private study to acquaint himself better with the writings of Cicero, Aristotle and Plato' was favoured by the fact that printing had already made books much more available for the individual student[1]; they had become more plentiful and less expensive and unwieldy. Gering, earliest of the Paris printers,

1 Cf. A. Tilley, *Studies in the French Renaissance*, p. 174.

advertised in one of his law books (*Corpus Juris Canonici*, vol. III) in 1500:

> Ne fugite ob pretium, dives pauperque venite:
> Hoc opus excellens venditur aere brevi.[1]

Aldus Manutius, the enlightened and progressive Venetian printer, had at the very opening of the century moved toward making the printed book less cumbersome. In Paris the Estiennes' press had followed him in this, and when, on the death of Henri Estienne, Simon de Colines, marrying the widow, took over, he too continued to move towards lessening the printed book's size and cost. Among manuals for the courses in Arts, the *Flores* of Mercarius would be exceptional in being of folio size. Other things equal, the smaller the format of a volume the less the cost, and therefore price to the student. Price lists of de Colines are still extant.[2] The 8° volume sold at 3–8 sols, the 4° at 10–12, the 2° at 15–25. The little 16°, developed by de Colines, was priced at only 3–5 sols. The law books were more refractory—they continued for the most part huge, and stuck to gothic type. But de Colines, with his pride in skilled typography, his famous Geoffrey Tory device and initials, and his artistic title-pages and woodcut illustrations, employed, like a good humanist, roman character—the 'humanist type' as it is sometimes called—and eschewed gothic so far as possible. All this was favourable to the needy student. Simon de Colines is thought to have succeeded Henri Estienne as a *messager* in the University; the office of *messager* took responsibility for certain expenses of those students who came from a distance. Such students were grouped for that purpose according to the diocese whence they came. The young Fernel would have been of the diocese of Amiens, and perhaps some relation of that sort between him and de Colines was a factor in the publishing of his earliest book at the famous Colines press, even before he had taken his M.D. degree. Fernel's own folios of 1527 and 1528 were priced at 5 sols, but with two at least of them went a companion volume of plates priced at 10 and 12 sols (Ph. Renouard).[3]

It was only when Fernel actually proceeded to the more advanced stage of scholarship on which he now entered that he realized how sadly his previous studies had gone awry. All he had done so far,

1 'Do not shy at the price: come, rich and poor. This admirable work is cheap.'
2 Bibliothèque Nationale.
3 Ph. Renouard, *Bibliographie des éditions de Simon de Colines, 1526–46*, Paris, 1894.

Plancy tells us, had been to pick up futilities from 'barbarian' tutors. 'He could perhaps take the situation more calmly because it was one which befell his fellow-students and himself alike, and was no fault of his own; it was a feature of the age he lived in. In truth, at that time the University of Paris, once the foremost in all the world since the beginning of things, was, in the matter of the Arts course, backward and "barbarian".'[1]

Plancy's 'Life' tells us how Fernel resolved

that the path he had missed he must now find, and follow with all his strength. To that end he denied himself entertainments, feasts, drinking-bouts, convivialities, and much even of the companionship of comrades and acquaintances. He took small account of food and sleep and proper exercise, of ailments and affairs; he sacrificed everything to making himself proficient in the true knowledge of the liberal arts. He devoted all that in him lay wholly to that one end, all his diligence, thought and toil. His sole satisfaction was letters and learning. He counted every hour lost which was not spent in reading the great authors. He was infatuated with learning. Among his first cares was to amend his latin style, and free it from barbarisms. Such barbarisms were a vice of the age; and he had acquired them from his unscholarly teachers.[2]

This indictment of the progressive Collège de Ste Barbe, and in the second decade of the sixteenth century, is somewhat surprising. Does not Plancy here make a mountain of some molehill? The stress he puts on the whole incident, and the space he devotes to it, within a brief biographical sketch, set us asking: Why should he so stress it? What really was the nature of the importance he attached to it? Its date was 1519. If we adopt Goulin[3] on the date of his birth, Fernel would then be twenty-two. Plancy speaks of his good progress in 'disputation' in the two years leading to his degree. The length of the course for the M.A. was usually four years. Therefore Plancy's charge of linguistic 'barbarism' in the Arts School in Paris applies to the latter half of the second decade of the new sixteenth century. His specific indictment against the University teaching at that time is 'its Grammarians and Rhetoricians had in their hands nothing but rude Alexanders, Theopagituses, *Graecismuses*, Theodoletuses and a ruck of writings of that stamp. Its Dialecticians taught from nothing but the *Termini* of Clichtoveus, the *Summulae* of Peter of

---

1 *Vita. V. infra,* Note II, *Appendix,* p. 150.   2 *Vita.*
3 Goulin. *V. infra,* Note VI, *Appendix,* p. 173.

Spain, the *Logica* of Bricotius, and other like works.'[1] This then was the head and front of the offending. After hearing it we may still feel puzzled at the seriousness it assumes in Plancy s eyes. Further consideration, I think, finds that the circumstance carries with it a broad significance at first not plain to us to-day, but to Plancy too obvious to require explanation.

The great movement, often known as the Renaissance, was already making headway in France at the time to which Plancy's account refers. It was active, not least in Paris. Its spearhead, so to say, was 'humanist scholarship', displacing medieval. But, over and above that, the movement stood for a new culture and outlook upon life. Plancy is saying that the University has not given the young Fernel his rightful entry into this new movement, nor his rightful chance of understanding and sharing the new spirit of the age. The young Fernel was contemporary with the new movement. Paris and the court were already astir with it. But the University? Why had not the University equipped its young scholar to participate in and be a living part of it? Plancy's charge was that the University did not change its 'miserable' type of scholarship, and had left its young M.A. unqualified for recruitment into the ranks of the new Letters. It had bolstered up a superannuated medievalism at the expense of the culture of its young alumnus. In short, the inwardness of the complaint brought by Plancy was that the University had withheld the Renaissance from its young M.A.

Francis I was on the throne, and, at his court, the French Renaissance was already in flower. The new spirit was already alive in letters, fine art, painting and architecture. But the Renaissance was not primarily a University movement. It was of extra-mural origin. Derived in the main from Italy, it centred eminently about certain princes, their entourage and courts. The University of Paris, with its Colleges and its medieval tradition, was slow to welcome change. It was for the most part against innovations. Moreover, the new movement was suspect of the Sorbonne and the strong Collège de Navarre. The Reuchlin controversy had shown that the new scholarship might be a nuisance in the shape of a higher criticism in divinity. The old bottle was unsuited for such new wine. Erasmus, at home in most places, yet was not so in the University of Paris. Nor after all was the University in certain matters undisputed mistress in its own house,

1 *Vita. V. infra*, Note II, *Appendix*, p. 151.

even as to letters and scholarship. In comparison with Mother Church the University was still small and relatively upstart. Abbey and priory, at hand and afar, dwarfed it. Moreover, within the University itself the Church had its own fortress, the Sorbonne.

But the University had an asset of value; it possessed the personal patronage of the king. The crown had been becoming stronger, a stronger element in the new nationhood of France. Francis I cultivated his contacts with the University. Guillaume Budé, royal librarian at Fontainebleau, had the king's ear, and Budé was rated the finest humanist scholar of the time. In 1530, at the instance of Budé, Francis I was to found the 'Royal College' in Paris, with its Chairs of Greek and Hebrew, outposts of the new Letters, and of the Renaissance.

There had been an attempt as far back as 1470, abortive though it proved, to implant humanist scholarship into the University of Paris. At the Sorbonne itself, the librarian and the rector of that time, at their own charge, had imported two printers from Basle, and a press, and had set to work printing books for humanism. In a year's time, however, the rector had been called away to accompany a legation returning to Rome. The press, the earliest in France, had then moved from the Sorbonne, and gone to the rue St Jacques nearby. There it had given up printing 'humanism' because printing 'humanism' did not pay. The time to which Plancy's indictment of the University applies came forty-five years later, and by then the humanist movement in France had grown stronger. Further, the University quarter had become a hive of printing, centred on the rue St Jacques itself. In the matter of the printed book, Paris had come to rival Venice.

Plancy was, in his time, qualified to judge of scholarship. At Budé's death he was the pupil entrusted with editing the master's 'Epistles in Greek'. Part of Plancy's fulmination against the Faculty of Arts dealt with the grammars and manuals of rhetoric maintained in authority by the University in 1515–19. The new Scholarship took grammar and rhetoric very seriously. The two subjects were no longer mere lessons in memorizing maxims for divinity. Grammar and rhetoric were become living factors in good scholarship; without them there was no exact interpretation of the classics of literature. They had become elements in humanism—humanism, the fundamental factor in all human progress, if humanism itself was to be believed. As to the alleged superannuation of the books which Plancy pilloried, the 'Alexander' was the *Doctrinale* of Alexander of Villa-

Dei near Avranches, a latin grammar of the thirteenth century. It was in hexameter verse for ease of memorization. It had been in use already for three hundred years. During most of that period there would have been, in some schools, for a class using it, perhaps only one copy, the teacher's. At school the boys would learn to repeat it aloud. But printing had altered that situation.[1] The *Theodoletus* mentioned by Plancy appears also to have been an antiquated set of hexameters in latin, for the most part rhymed. The *Graecismus* likewise, despite its name, was a latin grammar, but it had a chapter dealing with elementary greek and containing a number of speculative greek etymologies. It too dated from the early thirteenth century; it was the compilation of Eberhard of Béthune. It may have been dictated to Erasmus when he was a schoolboy at Gouda or Deventer.

It would seem too, implementing further Plancy's accusation, that grammar and rhetoric received at this time very stepmotherly treatment from the University. Their teachers were not eligible to be regents. Their lectures were restricted to one hour a day, and that an hour following the midday meal. But in the new Scholarship these subjects had come to occupy key positions. Rhetoric, in the 'revival of letters', chose Cicero, especially the *Orations*, for its model. The Church was beginning to fear that Cicero as a moralist threatened to oust the Fathers.

As to dialectic and logic, Plancy's stricture names Peter of Spain, Bricotius and Clichtoveus. The *Summulae logicales* of Peter of Spain had in medieval times long been a favourite manual. It dated from the thirteenth century. Its authorship was uncertain; it had come to be attributed to the Spanish divine, elected Pope as John XXI. Whoever its author, the humanist movement found its versions of Aristotle very incorrect; and matters had not been improved by successive commentators. Again, Bricot, author of another *Logica*, was a glossarist of Aristotle, more recent than Peter of Spain, but still of medieval type. Rabelais satirized him by including imaginary works by him in the burlesque Library of St Victor. Rabelais bracketed him with Tartaretus, the well-known Aristotelian commentator ridiculed by Pierre Ramus, whose works were nevertheless reissued and reissued in the Paris of Fernel's student-time.

1 Richard Pynson's woodcut of a schoolroom, in the 'Oxford' latin grammar (printed in London, 1500), depicts three books among the eight schoolboys: *Informatio puerorum*, 4°.

That Plancy should condemn, in the same breath with Peter of Spain[1] and Bricot, his own contemporary Clichtoveus is less easily understandable. Jossé Clichtowe[2] was a favourite pupil of, and a collaborator with, Lefèvre d'Étaples, and Lefèvre is reputed one of the progressive influences making for humanism in France. Clichtowe, assisting Lefèvre in lecturing and writing, had contributed to the reaction against scholasticism and to the rise of humanism in France. His *Termini*, which Plancy arraigns, were two manuals, digests of Aristotelian logic, first published in 1505. One of them, *Fundamenta logica*, ran into eleven editions by 1560, nine of them issued in Paris. *Precipue in currentem logicen introductoria*, it claimed to be an up-to-date student manual for dialectic in the University of Paris, and as such it lived on, after the death of its author, actually into the time at which Plancy was writing this condemnation of him, somewhere between 1558 and 1567. The other *Termini* by Clichtowe gained even greater popularity; a larger volume, it went through eighteen editions between 1505 and 1535. As a student Fernel may have used it. Among its publishers was Henri Estienne, the humanist printer. Besides dialectic, it included grammar and rhetoric. It defines rhetoric as 'persuading by words' and logic as 'separating true from false'. Lefèvre, a liberal catholic and a pioneer of French humanism, and Budé, also a liberal catholic and a leader of French humanism on its actual arrival, were friends, as well as humanist allies. Clichtowe, trusted pupil of Lefèvre, and Plancy, trusted pupil of Budé, should, one would have expected, have been allies. One would suppose that as literary contemporaries in Paris they would be personally acquainted and sympathetic with each other. But Plancy's reference to Clichtoveus' popular text-book suggests antagonism. There was considerable difference of age, there may have been religious estrangement. Goulin (1775) refers to Clichtowe as one of the most famous theologians. The point is worth raising if it can throw light on Fernel's own position in religion, in a time and a society torn by growing religious passion. Plancy's Preface in his posthumous edition of Fernel (1567) makes bitter reference to the religious warfare around him. Both the Preface and his 'Life' of Fernel show Plancy to have been a man of strong feeling and temperamental nature. That is a difference between his Preface and any of Fernel's own. Fernel seems

1 André Thevet (1584) similarly brackets together Clichtoveus' *Termini* and Peter's *Summulae* as impeding reform of scholarship in the University.

2 *V. infra*, Note III, *Appendix*, p. 171.

remote from faction, alike in regard to State, Religion and Faculty. The nearest he manifests to dislike in his printed works is perhaps to Avicenna, the nearest to personal regard is to Henri II, both when dauphin and when king. From his association with Simon de Colines and then with Christian Wechel as publishers, it would seem that he was 'liberal' in his religious views. But Luther, as almost an antithesis to Humanism, would not be to his taste. Fernel's appointment to the court—where popular opinion associated him particularly with the cure of Catherine de Medici, and again of Diane de Poitiers, both of them strongly opposed to the 'Reformed Church' party—indicates that he was certainly not openly identified with the reform party. On the other hand, Le Paulmier, an assistant and secretary to him for some time, is said [1] to have suffered imprisonment at one period, as a dissident from the Church. And we cannot suppose Guillaume Plancy, living in his household for ten years, and his personal pupil and intimate assistant, to have held religious views strongly opposed to Fernel's own. Plancy, we have to think, was of 'liberal' view in religion, even as was his master Budé, under whom he had learned to be a scholar—Budé who had not hesitated to emend, in places, the text of the Vulgate itself. Plancy's lament, in the Preface (1567),[2] over the religious violence of the time may well be taken as a plea for tolerance. 'A Frenchman and an Englishman who hold the same religion have more kindness and friendship for one another than two citizens of the same town who differ in this respect', said l'Hôpital, Chancellor of France, in the year 1561. André Wechel, the printer of the *Universa Medicina* containing Plancy's Preface, became himself, shortly afterward, a fugitive from France to escape persecution for

1 Wickersheimer, *Les Médecins en France à l'époque de la Renaissance*, 1906.
2 There is a poem*, published in Lyons in the year of Plancy's Preface, on the state of France:

> ...... urbes orbas generosis civibus, agros
> Destitui cultore, uxorem conjuge, fratrem
> Germano, patrem nato, natum patre, portum
> Merce, vias obsessas furibus, arma vigere,
> Jus vinci, regem subigi, etc....

Cf. Note IV, p. 171. The contemporary engravers Tortorel and Périssin depicted these scenes.

* (Insidiosae Pacis Dissuasio, ad Carolum Nonum Galliarum Regem Christianissimum, Leodegario à Quercu Authore. Lugduni. Apud Benedictum Rigaudum, 1567. cum permissione. Apud viduam P. Attaignant in vico Citharae, prope templum divi Cosmae. 8°.)

religion—that is, he was identified with the Reformed Church party. We cannot think it probable therefore that Plancy had leanings towards the Catholic League.

Now Jossé Clichtowe, on the other hand, was notoriously an opponent of the Reformed Church party. On the question of celibacy of the clergy he, as publicist, attacked Erasmus. The dedication of his commentary (Paris, 1513)[1] on the *Theologia* of John the Damascene, the text by Lefèvre d'Étaples, opens with 'nothing ought to be more assured or fixed for us than the rescripts, rules and articles of the Catholic Faith, and we should all assent to them, without either hesitation or appeal to reason [rationis efflagitatione]'. We can imagine the scholium of Erasmus on this! Jossé Clichtowe, long a member of the Sorbonne, died a canon of Chartres. There may well have been antagonism between Plancy and Clichtowe on the ground of religion.

The cultural mishandling of the young Fernel by the University of Paris would therefore be, legitimately enough, a large mis-demeanour in the eyes of his devoted younger disciple Plancy, himself a humanist. Plancy would likely enough have been a sym-pathizer among the audience when Pierre Ramus gave, in 1546, the memorable address[2] on reform of the studies of the University of Paris. The culture of the young Fernel had been, Plancy would say, sacrificed to bolster up a decaying medievalism in the University. It is clear however, from Plancy's account, that the young M.A., surrounded by Paris, soon came to realize for himself the heavy mishap which had befallen his education. Plancy does not tell us how he came to do so. All he says is—and it is a remarkable story—that the young Fernel, giving up immediate prospects, decided, cost what it might, to turn back in his academic tracks and, despite the applause he had won, begin afresh and pick up, step by step, the new Scholarship. The intense earnestness with which, Plancy tells us, he did this shows him moved as by a fresh ideal in life. He plunged into the recasting of his studies as if into a tide of revivifying self-enlighten-ment. There was in him both enthusiasm and revolt. It was as a humanist he was lecturing on philosophy publicly at Ste Barbe at

[1] Haec Damasceni cū expositione prima aemissio typis absoluta est Parisiis ex officina Henrici Stephani e regione Scholae Decretorum Anno Christi omniū cōditoris et rectoris M.D.XII, nonis Februariis. Theologia Damasceni quatuor libris explicata.

[2] *De studiis philosophiae et eloquentiae conjungendis:* also *Præmium reformandae parisiensis accademiae* addressed to Charles IX.

the age of twenty-nine (A. Thevet, 1584).[1] Some words which he was to write ten years later suggest themselves here as context: 'Not to swerve from the old path of our forefathers! What if they had never swerved? No; it has been good for philosophy to move into fresh paths; against the voice of the detractor, against the dead weight of tradition, and against the fullness of ripe authority. So shall each age grow its own crop of new authors and new arts.'[2]

As for a career it would seem that, at this date, Fernel had no particular career in mind. He became, for a time, just a recluse, reading 'humane letters', and studying, along with them, some mathematics. This way of life, unremittingly pursued for more than five years, brought him to the age of twenty-seven, and to the year 1524. It would seem also to have been—and that does not surprise us—a period of recasting his taste and views, although spent chiefly amid books and private pupils.

Then a quartan fever laid him by. He had to leave Paris for the country-side, and fresh air. Recovery was slow. The question of a career then forced itself on him. Before him, according to Plancy, lay Church, Law or Medicine. He thought things over and consulted friends. He chose Medicine. It would seem (Plancy) that he thought the Church too great a plunge into affairs. The Law offered emolument, and social position, and his attainments in the liberal arts promised, so his friends said, certainty of success. But the bustle of the courts was distasteful to him, and he knew himself slow in debate. He felt his natural disposition to be more that of a student. Moreover, adds Plancy, his severe illness had been a demonstration to him of the essential beneficence attaching to medicine. A doctorate in medicine required, however, a University curriculum of four further years. So far his father had contributed to keep him. His father now wrote that, in fairness to the other children, he could no longer do so. But Fernel held to his decision to enter upon medicine. He would support himself by teaching. Plancy tells us he gave public lectures, on philosophy, in the Collège de Ste Barbe, and that his lectures 'won praise from all'. His earliest book, published a little later, contains homage from four of his public pupils. Mathurin Cordier was, 1525–1528, among the lecturers at Ste Barbe. Cordier was active in the reform of the Arts courses. He was a humanist and educationalist, after the type of da Feltre and Guarino earlier in

1 *Les Vrais Pourtraits des Hommes Illustres.*
2 Condensed from Preface of book i of the 'Dialogue'.

13

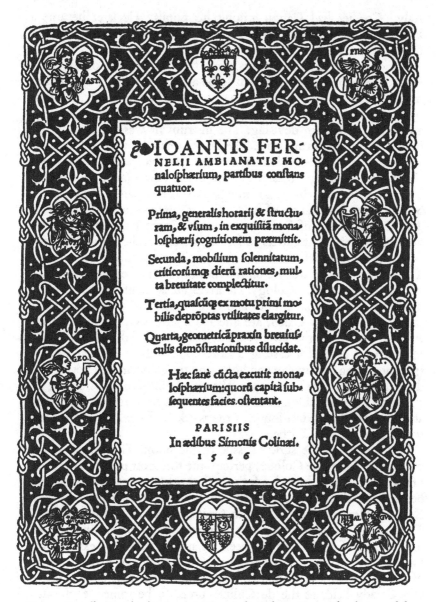

⁊◦IOANNIS FER-
NELII AMBIANATIS MO-
naloſphærium, partibus conſtans
quatuor.

Prima, generalis horarij & ſtructu-
ram, & vſum, in exquiſitã mona-
loſphærij cognitionem præmittit.

Secunda, mobilium ſolennitatum,
criticorúmq; dierũ rationes, multa breuitate complectitur.

Tertia, quaſcũq; ex motu primi mo-
bilis deprõptas vtilitates elargitur.

Quarta, geometricã praxin breuiuſ-
culis demõſtrationibus diſucidat.

Hæc ſanè dicta excutit mona-
loſphærium: quorũ capitã ſub-
ſequentes facies oſtentant.

PARISIIS
In ædibus Simonis Colinæi.
1 5 2 6

Fig. 2. Fernel's *Monalosphaerium*, 4°; Simon de Colines, Paris. The design of the border is attributable to Oronce Finé.

Italy. Cordier had Calvin among his pupils. He later became a
Protestant. Fernel and Cordier, teaching at the same College and at
the same time, would likely enough meet.

Plancy relates that about this time, that is, the time of his commencing medicine, Fernel began to be attracted specially to 'mathematics'. In the early spring of 1527, when he was thirty, his first
book[1] appeared and it was mathematical. It described a kind of
astrolabe of his own devising. The instrument was for finding the
hour and for measuring time. The book concludes with a discussion
of the days, and the divisions of the year. Its dedication, dated from
'the most famous gymnasium of Ste Barbe', is to Jacob de Govea,[2]
a mathematician, who was, though not at that time, Principal of
Ste Barbe, and was uncle of André Govea, also at one time Principal.
The Goveas were of Portuguese stock. Some latin verses in the
volume in praise of it and its author are by one of the author's pupils,
and there is homage from three other pupils, one of them Portuguese.
The work is a short treatise on the motions of the heavens. It shows
Fernel interested in astrology. It gives an account of the 'critical
days' and of the lunar month and of its medical bearings, and how
these last, to follow Galen, are affected by the signs of the Zodiac.
A table sets forth the twenty-eight mansions of the moon. Two
methods are given for casting a horoscope and are illustrated by a
specimen, for a certain day and hour, and the conventional horoscope
diagram is figured. The instance taken is 3 o'clock in the morning of
4 August 1526, which suggests the book was in course of being written
at that date. The dedication calls the work 'a fledgeling leaving the
warm nest', i.e. Ste Barbe.

Noteworthy is the style of issue of the book. The printer is no
other than Simon de Colines, perhaps the foremost printer in France
of that time. The volume is a folio, and its title-page carries a pictorial
border, the designing of which has been recently argued by Mr
E. P. Goldschmidt, to be due to Oronce Finé, the mathematician.
The large initial letters of the text, figurated and criblé, are themselves
little works of art. There has been no sparing either of expense or
pains in the production of the book, although the maiden work
of an unknown and poor man. It would seem that either Fernel
was already held, at the de Colines press, to be someone of out-

1 *Monalosphaerium. V. infra,* p. 187, Bibliog. 1.
2 Note V, *v. infra, Appendix,* p. 172.

standing promise, or that he had a generous patron at his back. With it was issued an album of figures of which no copy seems now extant.[1]

His second book followed in a year's time. Its title is *Cosmotheoria*, on the shape and size of the Earth; it was issued in similar form, again by Simon de Colines. It contains Fernel's measurement, from observations of his own, of a degree of meridian. Although this work was in part crude, he is remembered for it. It obtained a result in close agreement with that established by Jean Picard one hundred and forty years later.[2] Smith, in the *Rara Arithmetica*, writes: 'Among the French physicians of the sixteenth century, who devoted themselves to mathematics, the only one of great distinction is Fernel. His measure of the length of a degree of meridian was so satisfactory as to entitle him to a worthy place in the history of geodesy.'[3] In the same year followed his third treatise, *De Proportionibus*, again mathematical, and again from the press of de Colines, and in the same format. It describes the use and theory of fractions. It again seems to have been accompanied by an album of plates.[4]

Fernel took his licence to practise medicine in 1530, and his M.D. in the October of that year. He obtained a second class. Plancy's comment is that not lack of knowledge but lack of money kept him out of the first class. The remark makes it still less probable that Fernel himself met the expenses of the three finely produced folio volumes from de Colines' press.

Now, with medical practice in front of him, he settled in Paris, attracted says Plancy, by the opportunity it afforded for contact with men of varied learning, and so for furthering his own culture. It was at this time that he entered into an arrangement with Jacques Louis Destrebey, a grammarian and rhetorician of distinction, of the Collège de Rheims, next door to Ste Barbe.

1 Ph. Renouard, *Simon de Colines*, p. 428. Cf. Bibliography, *infra*, p. 188.

2 Jean Picard, *Mesure de la Terre*, Paris, 1671. In the last chapter he records the measurement by Fernel. Picard's triangulation took almost the same ground as Fernel's; it went from Malvoisine near Paris to Sourdon near Amiens. His book was translated into English by Richard Waller, F.R.S., and published in London (R. Roberts) in 1688. Waller was editor of Hooke's *Posthumous Works* and translator of the *Saggi del Accademia del Cimento*, Firenze, 1666, edited by Magalotti. See also Todhunter's *History of the mathematical theories of attraction and the figure of the Earth*, arts. 102, 236, 989, London, 1873.

3 *Rara Arithmetica*, D. E. Smith, Boston and London, 1908.

4 Ph. Renouard, *Simon de Colines*.

Their compact was for Fernel to give Destrebey tuition in mathematics in return for receiving tuition 'in the fine flower of classical letters' (Plancy). Destrebey was somewhat the older man. In the library of the British Museum there are four books by him: one a rhetoric in two editions (Paris, 1540; Lyons, 1541), one a commentary on Cicero's *Orations* (Paris, 1540) and a compendium of Quintilian, which reached a second edition, Paris, 1550. Sir Thomas Browne,[1] in the seventeenth century, cites Cicero's *Cato Major* in Destrebey's edition as a standard text. Plancy remarks a noticeable development in Fernel's latin style subsequent to the three mathematical tracts, and attributes this to Destrebey's instruction. 'Fernel's style gained in dignity and fullness from Destrebey.'[2]

Goulin,[3] in his biographical account of Fernel (1775), based on Plancy, suggests that Fernel probably did not read greek. He places that interpretation on Plancy's mention of Marsilio Ficino's latin rendering of Plato. Goulin would seem, however, to be mistaken in this inference. Plancy's prefatory letter, dedicating to Fernel his (Plancy's) latin version of Galen's *Aphorisms* of Hippocrates, remarks it may well be that Fernel will 'prefer to read the *Aphorisms* in their greek; but that the work is offered simply as a tribute by a pupil to his Master'.[4] Moreover, Fernel's practice, in the 'Pathology' and elsewhere, of furnishing his marginalia in greek, and also commonly, when desiring to define a term, resorting to a greek equivalent, for instance in his Preface to 'The Natural Part of Medicine', do not countenance the notion. That he did not read greek may be dismissed.[5]

Destrebey pursued letters as a humanist. The fact identifies Fernel further with the 'revival of letters' and the 'humanist movement'. A passage in Fernel's 'Dialogue'—which, for its sentiment, pleased more than two hundred and fifty years later the ear of the infant French Republic, in its 'year one'—has a typical Renaissance ring:

Many tell us that the art of healing, discovered by the labours of our forefathers, and brought to completion by dint of Reason, has now attained its goal. They would have us, who come after, tread in the same footsteps as did the Past. It were a crime, they tell us, to swerve a hair's breadth

1 *The Garden of Cyrus*; London, 1658; 8°, pp. 92, 94.   2 *Vita.*
3 *Mémoires littéraires, etc.*, Paris, 1775.
4 *Galeni in Aphorismos Hippocratis Commentarii VII.* Recens per Gulielmum Plantium Cenomanum; Lugd. 1552.
5 Cf. Note VI, *Appendix*, p. 174.

from the well-established way. But what if our elders, and those who preceded them, had followed simply the same path as did those before them?...Nay, on the contrary it seems good for philosophers to move to fresh ways and systems; good for them to allow neither the voice of the detractor, nor the weight of ancient culture, nor the fullness of authority, to deter those who would declare their own views. In that way each age produces its own crop of new authors and new arts. This age of ours sees art and science gloriously re-risen, after twelve centuries of swoon. Art and science now equal their ancient splendour, or surpass it. This age need not, in any respect, despise itself, and sigh for the knowledge of the ancients. The orator to-day attains the height of oratory. Philosophy excels in every branch. Once again music, geometry, the handicrafts, painting, architecture, sculpture, and many other kinds of skill display themselves in such measure as in no wise to fall short of the achievements of antiquity, which won universal praise.... Our age to-day is doing things of which antiquity did not dream. Antiquity held Demetrius high for his engines of war, but to-day we have petards which hurl a flaming bomb. Good God, how destructive and swift compared with the old catapult! How efficient to-day the printing-press for the diffusion of all kinds of learning. To-day we have paper, once called Fabriano,[1] supplanting wax, bark and skin. Hence 'letters' to-day reach their high-water mark. Ocean has been crossed by the prowess of our navigators, and new islands found. The far recesses of India lie revealed. The continent of the West, the so-called New World, unknown to our forefathers, has in great part become known. In all this, and in what pertains to astronomy, Plato, Aristotle, and the old philosophers made progress; and Ptolemy added a great deal more. Yet, were one of them to return to-day, he would find geography changed past recognition. A new globe given us by the navigators of our time. Over and above that a method of ascertaining what geographers term 'longitude', in whatever quarter of the globe.[2]

Plainly this is the Renaissance speaking, with what Hazlitt and Keats called 'the gusto of the Elizabethan voice'. The time was past when Roger Bacon would write: 'We, how do we compare with the ancients? We have discovered nothing worthy of those philosophers. We cannot even understand their wisdom.' Fernel's sentiments tell us that the long reign of that old inferiority complex is over. The Middle Ages, with their retrospective gaze, lie behind; the Renaissance, eager for to-day and to-morrow, is in possession. A new

1 From the early paper mills in Italy; the objection which paper had to meet was that it was more perishable. Louis XI had decreed that legal documents must not be on paper.
2 Preface to book i of the 'Dialogue'.

generation was abroad like boys just out of school. The time was
come of the great navigators. We see we can accept Fernel as
representing the Renaissance around him. He himself is undertaking
a work thirteen centuries had left unventured. To do so was in the
spirit of the age.

Fernel married[1] into a family of good and substantial position. His
father-in-law was a councillor of the 'Parlement' of Paris. Plancy,
as Bayle remarks, does not say of which court. The main professional
preoccupation of Fernel at this period seems to have been studying
the sky and stars. He had already written three tracts touching
that subject, and he had devised an astrolabe, a sort of precursor of
Oronce Finé's of the year following his. He now designed further
instruments; he even kept craftsmen in his house constructing and
engraving them. To meet their cost he dipped into his wife's dowry.
At length his father-in-law, a business-like man, expostulated. Fernel
could not, however, give it up. Finally open rupture with his family
threatened. There were tears from his wife and children, says Plancy.
Only then did Fernel at last consent to put his mathematics aside.
The craftsmen and engravers were dismissed, the costly bronze
instruments dismantled, his library of the old 'mathematicians' was
disposed of, and he told his pupils they must find their teaching in
that subject elsewhere. He turned all his energy to what we should
call medicine proper.

Why these mathematics? And what were they? They never saw
the light in print. What was the fascination in them? Plancy, Fernel's
pupil, remarks: 'Contemplation of the stars and heavens so astonishes
and charms the mind that we are taken in the toils of a delighted
bondage and become enslaved.'[2]

That, however, does not tell us what the studies were. Evidently
they involved the stars and costly instruments. Were they astrology?
Thevet mentions 'astrolabes' among the instruments. In the 'Life',
Plancy expresses strong disapproval of astrology. It seems significant
that the 'Life', which has something to say about each one of

1 Fernel's wife Madeleine was a Tournebulle. He had by his marriage two
children, daughters. They married men of some distinction. Some account of
them is given in one of Guy Patin's letters, Letter 61, written from Paris,
25 September, 1655, to Monsieur A.F.C.M.D.R. In the edition of the *Letters*,
Paris, 3 vols. 1692, the reference is vol. i, p. 169. Cf. also Fernel's posthumous
'Cure of Fever' (Bibliog. 95.M1), dedicated by J. Lamy to Jean Barjotte,
Seigneur of Marchefrai, grandson of Fernel.

2 *Vita. V. infra*, Note II, *Appendix*, p. 158.

Fernel's other works published in his lifetime, is silent about the three mathematical treatises, finely issued though they were, by the best printer in France, and marking the beginning of Fernel's whole career as a writer. Fernel, Plancy explains, though he thought that 'the astronomy which deals with the motions and revolutions of the heavens, and with the risings, courses, and settings of the stars, is of good use to the physician', came finally to look back with bitter regret on having, at one period of his life, cultivated astrology, and devoted much time to it.

Fernel, as a young physician, clearly enjoyed a reputation for his computations and his mathematics. 'Mathematicians' and 'astrologers' had long been put together by the public as of a class—so far back as St Augustine in his century, and Isidore of Seville in his. The public mind still regarded them as birds of a feather. It styled both of them 'mathematicians'. Gasparinus, in *De Eloquentia*, a compendium of latin phrases, with a foreword by that same Iodocus Clichtoveus of whom Plancy above was scornful, sets forth the terms suitable for addressing persons of various qualities and callings. Physicians, he says, are to be addressed *Mathematici, sapientes perspicacesque.*[1] It seems natural to connect Fernel's activity in mathematics in his early days with Plancy's statement of a phase in his life when he was greatly intrigued by astrology.

Fernel lived to disabuse himself of astrology. Plancy tells us so, and Fernel's own writings attest it. Following them, we can trace roughly the duration of his astrological pursuits. He had thrown them off largely by 1542, that is in twelve years' time from taking his doctorate in medicine, and fifteen years after the publication of his mathematical tractates. His treatise on 'Physiology' (1542) is altogether restrained as to astrology. The theme of the book is largely a theoretical examination of man the living creature, as introductory to the facts and theory of medicine. The theme could therefore, in the hands of a medical astrologer, have justified frequent references to astrology. But Fernel is circumspect, and, on the whole, markedly detached from astrology. In one problem, a problem of special difficulty for him and his time, he does indeed invoke unrestrainedly the occult and the stars, though not exactly in the form of astrology.

A further opportunity for gauging the author's attitude to astrology at that date is given in the general Preface with its discussion of what

---

1 Gathering h vii, verso: *De Eloquentia*, Paris, 8°.

medicine is, what its rank as knowledge, and what kinds of learning it requires. An enthusiast in medical astrology would there, we may think, have taken the opportunity to show his astrological learning and leanings. But Fernel does neither. The passage is of interest in several ways. Fernel arranges knowledge and vocation in a scale of worthiness. Highest stand philosophy and theology, 'treating of the gods'; then mathematics, which likewise treats of eternal things; thence descending by history, geography, dialectics, rhetoric, architecture to the purely utility accomplishments, the crafts, such as the gold-worker's, the weaver's, the butcher's, the painter's, the scribe's, and ultimately, with nice particularity, to the flute-player's, the dancer's, the cook's, the sausage-stuffer's, the pimp's, and the gamester's, who purvey merely for our grosser pleasures—some of them unworthy and even vicious ones. Finally, as to medicine, he asks: 'Is there a greater blessing vouchsafed to mankind than Medicine is? Life is our dearest possession, by which we breathe and enjoy the company of our fellow-beings. Can any calling be worthier than that which preserves and maintains life itself? Is wealth or fortune, in whatever measure, in the last resort, more estimable than is good health? Is any misfortune or disaster more grievous than ill-health? He who succours the sufferer and the sick exercises a knowledge which deserves the admiration and affectionate regard of all men'[1] (abridged). This forecasts in our time Carlyle's 'the physician can abolish pain, relieve his fellow-mortals from sickness. He is indisputably usefullest of all men.' Fernel's statement here can be taken in some sort as a gloss on Plancy's account of why Fernel chose medicine for his calling.

Fernel then goes on to mention the various sorts of knowledge required by the physician. It ranges from grammar and rhetoric to the 'stars in their courses'. The physician must be adept too in the material and procedures medicine employs. Cicero, he says, did not esteem learning *in vacuo*, or the mere contemplation of Nature. Knowledge is to be assessed by its practical value. It must be useful for something. Lacking that, it is superfluity and vanity. The painter, besides painting the picture, has to prepare the panel and grind the pigments. He must, as Aristotle says, 'know all the means toward his end.'[2] Social service is often a motive with Fernel. The 'Pathology'

1 *Praefatio*, called in the collected works by the Heurnes the 'General Preface to the Medicine' (Bibliog. 86.J30).
2 *Praefatio*.

has a foretaste of the eugenics of to-day. 'These beginnings of our being are therefore of much matter to us. Those of us who are endowed with health in virtue of our birth are not a little fortunate. It would be a great good for our race if solely those who are sane and sound gave themselves to the making of children. The husbandman knows that in sowing the land the best seed is to be chosen. Experience

Vàm illæ variè comparari foleant: ęstimari certò non antè poteſt, quàm figillatim cuiuſque vires quãtæ ſint expenderimus. Auerrhoïs vt eſt in omnes ferè contu- melioſus, ſic & Galenu erroris falſò inſimulauit, quòd ſummas elementorum qualites in temperatione haberi cenſuerit. Hęc dum paucis immutatis corrigere vult, omnia deprauaſſe vide- ri poteſt, qui tum ſpecies, tum qualitates elemétorum ad mediocre quiddã in concretione retundi reprimíque putat. In illa formarum remiſſione quãtum ſit lapſus, perpéſum à nobis alio loco eſt. Nunc verò ſi qualitates ſummas in confuſionem quandam adductas, ait ſeſe mutuò poſſe ad mediocritatem deducere, cur non ſimiliter ſeſe prorſus interimunt? Sunt ſanè media hæc vtl & ſumma inter ſeſe contraria. Scio opinationem quandam apud neotericos peruulga-

Contra Auer- rhoïdem,

Dialogorũ li. j.
Ratio prima.

Fig. 3.

De quibuſcunque ratio, de eiſ dem & imaginatio delirat.	Adem nomina gene- rum & partium ani-
216.a	mæ. 127.b
De ſcroto obſeruatio 33.b	Effigies. 255.b
Dialogorum Ioan. Ferne. lib.	Eiuſdem partis animæ ſunt
i. 90.a	imaginatio, & memoria.
Diaphragma 35.b	214.b
Differentiæ parenchy. 63.a	Electio. 151.b.212.b

Fig. 4.

Figs. 3, 4. References in the 1st edition, 1542, and in the 2nd edition, 1547, of the *De Naturali Parte Medicinae* to the 'Dialogue' not then printed.

has taught him that from poor seed he can expect only a miserly harvest. How much more strictly should that precept be practised in the propagation of our species?'[1] This passage rang novel in its time. It is quoted by Robert Burton as such, even in the following century, in his *Anatomy of Melancholy*.[2]

Returning to Fernel's Preface, its allusion to astrology is slight and

1 *Pathol.* i, c. 11.　　　　　　2 Burton abounds in references to Fernel.

even equivocal, for it may mean astronomy proper, not astrology. 'Medicine', it says, 'examines what is dug from the bared bowels of the earth, and, turning on high, observes the wheelings of the heavens and the forces flowing and spreading thence which control this lower sphere'[1]—a statement succinct and restrained, compared with some pronouncements in his earlier writings.

In the 'Hidden Causes', the 'Dialogue', as he called it, there is much more of astrology and the occult than in the 'Physiology'. Evidence is clear that the 'Dialogue' was written the earlier;[2] cf. also Prof. L. Thorndike, *History of Magic and Experimental Sciences*, Vol. v.

The 'Physiology' was first printed in 1542, and in that, its earliest edition, Fernel mentions in some of its marginals the 'Dialogue', and refers the reader to it, though it was not then printed. The second edition of the 'Physiology', printed in 1547, does so too, and even items 'Fernel's Dialogues' in its index. The 'Dialogue' was therefore regarded as accessible to the readers of these early editions of the 'Physiology'. And the writing of the 'Physiology' dates back in part to 1538, for, as Goulin[3] points out, it mentions[4] the execution of an assassin as taking place at the time it was being written, and the date of that execution is known to have been August 1538. The existence of the 'Dialogue' in MS. may therefore date back to ten years before its appearance from the press. Fernel states, in the Preface to the 'Dialogue', that the work had been written some long time, but had been withheld from more general circulation lest it be misconstrued by the larger public.[5]

The 'Dialogue' is therefore the earlier, and it shows Fernel interested in magic and astrology sufficiently to discuss their several aspects. Its author was then far from the point where, as in the *De Vacuundi Ratione* (1545), he dismisses astrology with the brief sentence: 'These common-sense rules are of more use than is astrological observation.'[6]

To appreciate this rejection by Fernel of astrology (and to a large extent of the occult as a whole) we must look at him in the setting of his time. In the mid-sixteenth century medicine was, taken generally, still under the influence of astrology and the occult; they

1 *Praefatio.*   2 See Note VI, *Appendix*, p. 174.

3 *Mémoires*, p. 298.   4 In the part dealing with ligaments, book i.

5 The 'Dialogue' evoked two commentaries. One by Jacques Aubert, *Progymnasmata in Johan. Fernelii libros de abditis rerum causis*, 1579; the other by Jean Riolan the Elder, *Ad libros Femelii de abditis rerum causis*, appearing first in 1589, dedicated to Philippe Muraults, reissued (1598) by H. Perier, 8°, Paris.

6 Cap. 16, repeated in the *Medicina* (1554), 'Therapeutics', book ii, c. 13.

were superstitions widely current. Medicine as we now watch it at work, rational and effective in the community, was not yet really on its feet. The scientific certitudes of modern medicine barely begin until the seventeenth century. What the heart was doing, what the blood was doing, why we take breath, were all mysteries unsolved—unguessed even to the extent that the existing ignorance did not suspect they were unsolved, or indeed regard them as mysteries at all. Nor did the unsuspecting Renaissance turn its mind to solving them. They were no concern of the new 'humanism'. They were to require an altogether new path of enquiry.

The art of healing had descended the Middle Ages beset by diffi-culties partly special to itself. For one thing, its organization, as beside that of its two elder contemporaries, Church and Law, was scanty and lax. Church and Law were organized like armies of occupation. They commanded every going and coming which could affect their interests. Such rules and conformity as they might decree, they could enforce. But Medicine had neither the system nor the powers. Its prestige was equivocal, attaching rather to an individual than to his cloth. Medicine went often flouted in the market-place. The preamble to a statute of the third year of our Henry VIII, that is when Jean Fernel was a lad of fifteen, tells something of this: 'Foras-much as the science and cunning of physic and chirurgy is daily exercised by multitudes of ignorant persons, so far that common artificers as smiths, weavers and women boldly and customarily take upon them great cures of things of great difficulty, in the which they use sorcery and apply medicines very noyous, to the displeasure of God, infamy to the faculty and grievous hurt to the king's liege people[1] most especially of them that cannot discern the uncunning from the cunning', and so on.

1 This preamble is a little reminiscent of that of the Edict of Philip the Fair of France, which instituted the College of 'sworn surgeons of Paris' in 1311. The king enacts that none shall exercise surgery 'in our city and county of Paris' until he has been examined by sworn surgeons summoned by the royal surgeon of the Châtelet and have taken an oath before the Chief Magistrate, because 'it has come to our notice that surgical treatment is being undertaken by many undesirables, some of them murderers, thieves, coiners of false money, rascals (holerii), cozeners, adventurers, alchemists (arquemistae) and userers, whose ignorance turns small wounds into mortal ones', etc. Punishment, prison until a fine is paid. (Reissue of 1644, printed as evidence for an appeal by the Royal College of Surgeons of Paris in that year. A similar preamble is employed in confirmation of this edict right on into Fernel's own times.)

Sorcery and magic were ingredients in this welter; and they were accredited very reputably. The fame of the poet Virgil was great as a magician rather than as a poet. Fulgentius Placitus found the *Georgics* a tissue of recipes for magic; Fernel himself hardly otherwise, in references to it in the 'Dialogue'. It was as magician that the poet had conducted Dante through hell and purgatory to paradise. 'Virgil the Sorcerer, treating of the Life of Virgilus, and of his death, and many Marvayles that he dyd in hys lyfe tyme by Whychcrafte and Nygramancye through the help of the devyls of Hell' was a book[1] new in Fernel's own time. The age looked on natural magic as a thing as assured as medicine itself. To exercise magic was part of the rôle of the physician.

Another factor in the mystification was astrology. The Church did restrain sorcery, but to restrain astrology was beyond the Church's strength. 'At Rome', said Savonarola, writing about the year Fernel was born, 'no prelate, no rich man, but has at hand an astrologer to say whether he should ride forth or do anything. No one takes a step in life unless authorized by his astrologer.'[2]

Astrology was not in the general opinion necessarily opposed to religion. Some of the faithful accepted it as a sort of 'natural religion', with its place accessory to and alongside of the religion of the Church. A measure of learning was needed for its due comprehension. It appealed to the cultured perhaps more than to the populace. As to its contact with medicine, its argument contributed to medical theory and routine. Fernel's early tracts had been written to facilitate its computations for that purpose. Even at the time of writing his 'Hidden Causes', more sceptical than formerly of magic and astrology though he had then become, he gives to the character which impersonates himself the name of an old-time mathematician whom his text speaks of as 'astrologer'. Society, especially society of liberal view—and Fernel was a humanist and of the party of reform in the Faculty—inclined to see in medical astrology the Medicine with promise for the future, the climax of medical science. The questionable in it was less the astrological itself, than the personal competence or probity of this or that individual astrologer. Even as late as Diderot astrology was among what the 'Encyclopedia' called 'the respectable prejudices'.

1 London, 1550, 4°, ?W. Copland, in the British Museum.
2 Villari, *Storia di G. Savonarola*, I, p. 169.

An ancient system of knowledge and speculation, astrology drew authority from the past. The new scholarship of Fernel's time was busy with some of its texts. Astrology was not altogether outside humanism. Cardan of Milan, Fernel's acquaintance, was preparing a new commentary on the *Quadripartitae*[1] of Ptolemy, when he and Fernel met in Paris. The Chaldeans of pagan antiquity, equally with Arnald of Villanova, counsellor of fourteenth-century popes, had reckoned with this divination by the stars. Arabian science had perfected its calculations. Nightly throughout Christendom and Islam the astrolabes refined the observations further. It was an age when the eager-minded Cardan could declare, 'that the Earth moves is as impossible as that the heavens stand still'. The world in general was still deceived by that great sense-illusion, which lets us think we walk a stationary earth, while sun and stars sweep round us. Although naïve, it was soul-compelling. Its corollary was that our place is at the centre of the universe. The heavens like a ninefold shell enfolded us at its heart. They faced inward on us. What could it all mean, except that the *raison d'être* of it all was man? All else drew meaning from man. It was around man that the stupendous cavalcade of the zodiac paraded. Man himself was a microcosm, epitomizing his surround, the macrocosm. He and his surround acted and reacted, each on the other. To study man apart from the heavens was idle if we were to understand him. Fernel had spent nights with the stars; they formed the scene of his first free-lance adventure after know-ledge. The heavenly bodies, except sun and moon, were still but shining points. To Fernel, trusting observation as he did, the likeliest way to learn the effect of the stars on the sick man was to observe events in the two taken together, the one in the skies, the other in the sick-room.

There was, for example, the influence of the moon upon the drawing of blood. Fernel respected his forerunner Arnaldus, the physician of some three hundred years earlier—a first-hand observer, with views on fermentation. Listening over the shoulder of Arnaldus[2] we can hear his talk upon the blood at a blood-letting, an opportunity such as Fernel himself was wont to take:

There, you see, near the bottom of the pipkin, is the black bile, the melancholy, dark and earthy. Do not however suppose it wholly evil.

1 Printed at Basle, 1554.
2 A good edition of Arnaldus' collected works is that of Fradin, Lyons, 1504.

It is part of our fourfold cardinal nature. It is to nourish the melancholy organs, which are solid and cool, the bones, and even the spleen. It thickens and fortifies the blood. Excess of it is a disease. Yet there are those whom we regard rightly as healthy, who have, all their life, some excess of the black-bile. They make a type which the physician must recognize; disease in them takes character from that modicum of excess. They are sallow and dark and spare. They are solitary and taciturn, suspicious and sad. The 'melancholic' sums them up. On them certain of our medical herbs act with especial power. The melancholy humour remains through all its fermentations an enemy to joy, an ally of age and death. Those who have excess of it are supersensitive to certain phases of the moon, to certain conjunctions of the planets, to Saturn, and to certain houses of the zodiac.[1] The rich have it even as the poor. There is no difference between the blood in rich and poor. [Arnaldus had written a *Treasure of the Poor*.[2]] The planet which acts most on the four qualities of man is the moon, in its first quarter warm and moist, in its second, dry and warm; in its third, cold and dry, in its fourth, moist and cold. With each moon therefore for the first 7 days the blood dominates; then for 7 days the yellow bile, the choler; then for 7 days the black bile, the melancholy; and then the phlegm. From the moon's phases the crisis of an illness can be foretold. The moon's phase can enhance or interfere with a remedy. So it comes that measures can be taken which otherwise would avail nothing. One phase is good for blood-letting, another not.

But a further factor is the patient's elemental composition, his 'temperament'. Also, the organ itself is a factor to be considered. The sun rules the heart, the moon rules the brain, and the moon— Polixenes' 'watery star' in *The Winter's Tale*—is especially potent in woman; woman is the more moist, the more pituitous. The moon, ruling the brain, influences the mind. Its light, flooding a sleeper, can perturb the mind—yet the moon's light being reflected from the sun, some moonlight is benign. Toward all this, and toward much more which was akin to it, the earnest physician of Fernel's time had to orientate his conscience and his practice.

Would it seem fantastic to Fernel? There was nothing in it he would judge 'fantastic', or even perhaps extravagant. It was an

1 'Thus, the 7th is called the house of death' (*septimam mortis domum astronomi nominant*); S. Paparella, *De Calido*, i, c. xi, p. 34 r., Perusiae, 4°, 1573. But see below, Adam Wirdung. I have a MS. horoscope-schema of 1513 which inscribes the 8th house 'mortis'.

2 Guy de Chauliac remarks of it, 'I have not fully accepted or endorsed the empiricisms and enchantments of which I find in it a goodly number': *La Grande Chirurgie*, p. 598, edition of 1598.

adventure of thought, sanctioned and familiar from of old, and now
remoded. The intelligentsia has often developed a taste for endorsing
such ventures. Thus, there were the publications, much in vogue in
the time of Fernel, the ephemerides or calendars. We can choose one
of date 1556, two years after Fernel's latest instalment of his *Medicina*
and two years before his death. A small quarto of sixty-eight pages,
it describes itself as calculated by Bartholomaeus Reysacher, of
Carnten, Professor of Mathematics in the University of Vienna, with,

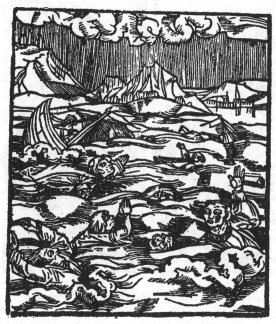

Fig. 5. From a *Practica* of 1521, illustrating the great flood predicted for 1524.

of course, the privilege of the emperor. Following each leaf of the
calendar proper is a blank page for MS. notes. The work is dedicated
to Sigismond, Freiherr of Herbeston. Our copy bears, written in on
its first blank, the names of the heads of the family, and of their
children at that date; the same hand has entered notes on many of the
blank pages. The calendar uses printed symbols, affixed to each day,
denoting the day as astrologically good, or moderately good, or
bad, for blood-letting, for purging, or for taking a bath, or again
showing whether the moon will be of evil light or favourable. Some
of the blanks are crowded with MS. notes. After the calendar follows

the *Practica* with its prognostications of diseases, etc., to be rife in the coming year. There are to be two eclipses and their astrological significance is set out, with figures of the occultations in woodcut. A whole page woodcut is given to the 'zodiac man', or 'anatomy', and indicates on him the places of election for bleeding under the twelve signs of the Zodiac.

In short the little book, German of the sixteenth century, stands

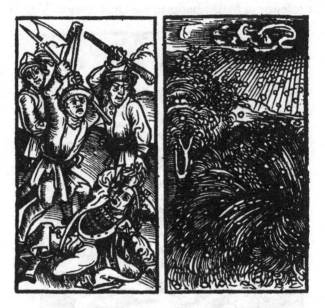

Fig. 6. From a *Practica* of 1521, illustrating its prophecy of
war and storm for 1524.

witness to superstition typical of its place and time. Carinthia, its particular locality, listened greedily to Theophrastus the 'paracelsus'.

From not far away, not much earlier, had come another *Practica* which in its time had made a stir; that of *mathematicus* Adam Wirdung, of Hassfürt, in the diocese of Würzburg. It had been printed first in latin, and then in the vernacular at Oppenheim (1521). Its preface is addressed to the Reverend Dr, both of Canon and Civil Law, Wernher of Themar. It claims the patronage of the new Emperor, Charles V, and of the elector Ludwig of the Rhenish Palatinate. The preface, written from Heidelberg, the ducal seat, is dated from the University there. Its pages announce a terrible new Conjunction, or

Assembling of Planets, for the approaching year, 1524.[1] A chart, drawn up somewhat after the manner of a horoscope, illustrates how, following the motion of the heavens, this Conjunction will ensue. Saturn, Jupiter and Mars, with Saturn evilly dominant, will meet in the 8th 'house of Heaven', the House of Death, under the watery sign, Pisces. This will happen 'by the laws of Plato in the book called *Thimeus*'. The year 1524 will be catastrophic, though, it is hoped, not without some reliefs. There will be a flood which will submerge the mountains nearly to their tops, but it will not be general—not a second Deluge, because of God's rainbow. But towns and castles will be drowned, there will be pestilence, and stars will fall like fiery dragons, and a comet with a tail which stretches out to far places will traverse the 12 signs. The just shall suffer, the old law be changed, and many shall die for their faith: and there shall be war and death among kings. The elements shall hinder the corn and the wine; no twig shall remain in the vineyard, and the corn shall be as good as ungrown; and many people shall starve. We must raise our eyes to heaven and pray lest our children and we die along with even the unreasoning beasts of the field. There will be unexampled war among the peoples. A hard and cruel people shall rise up, showing neither mercy nor pity; and shall kill, with cannon and weapons, old and young. They shall spare neither maid nor fruitful wife. The ground shall be cumbered with slain and with swords and weapons; and town and village be laid waste. Castle and hall and house shall be wrecked and burned. The slaughter shall drench the soil with blood, and nowhere shall a man know whither to turn from his foes. The people of low degree and baser sort will rise against king and noble, and persecute them miserably as under a similar Conjunction in the year of the world 2484. The nobles and the Kings shall buckle on their arms for vengeance.

1 Professor Lynn Thorndike (*History of Magic and Experimental Science*, vol. v, ch. xi) gives a chapter (pp. 178–232) to some of the circumstances of this 'conjunction of 1524'. He finds its literature includes 56 authors and 133 editions (G. Hellmann, *Beitr. Geschichte d. Meteorologie*, 1914). Thorndike traces the discussion to a Paris astrological tract, March 1519, by Albert Pigghe of Kampen, Holland, student of mathematics and theology.

Wirdung (*Allgem. Deutsch. Biographie*, 40, p. 9) was called by Christian II of Denmark to explain 'Genesis' to him. He died *c.* 1550. Professor Lynn Thorndike has written on him (see *History of Magic and Experimental Sciences*, v, 203 footnote), and adds (*H. of M. and E.S.* v, 203, 1941), 'I have some further MS. data as yet unpublished'. He gives some account of the *Practica* on pp. 203–4.

The change in the four qualities (of Hippocrates and Avicenna) owing to the change in the four seasons will bring illness to men and women, and young and old, and even to the beasts of the field. There shall be pestilential fever and disease of all parts of the body. As in the year of our Lord 1464 the Jews will be martyred, sold and punished so that they shall wail and cry aloud 'we have sinned'. Saturn with his dragon's tail will in some measure have strength to shield them, so that they are not wholly exterminated; many, to escape the worst, will be baptized. Under these Conjunctions the faithful of Christ themselves shall be imperilled and diminished. They shall drink the cup of bitterness at the hands of the base, the knave and the robber. The priest and prelate shall be at the mercy of the cut-throat, the house of prayer be like to become a house of gambling and a den of robbers.

There will be fighting against the Turk and the shedding of much Christian blood. The Saracens shall suffer, their dwellings shall be burnt, they shall feel the whip of God. As for Rome, let it remember the old prophecy, 'Woe to thee, Italy, woe to thee'. A great armed host of the well-born and the strong shall come from the north and lay low all Liguria and Italy, and burn town and castle and tower. And you, knights of Rome, sigh for your nobility overcome and for a great one who shall die in prison. And the growth and the fruit of the earth shall be destroyed and the sea shall drown much and many. France, take heed lest a foreign nation destroy you and bring you under subjection, and a German rule you in your pride, and the eagle nest in the lilies. Let England tremble, lest the wild animals devour the English people; they shall suffer disease and death and die in want. Scotland shall weep, for the sea shall do frightful harm to her, and her enemies shall cause her manifold woes; and diseases be rife. In Sweden the King will at last rule his people. Of the Bohemian people great numbers will turn to the Church of Rome and forsake their heresy and disbelief of the last hundred and 6 or 7 years.[1] But many nations shall gather together against the Bohemians and they can hardly escape great harm and woe. O Rhodes, awake lest the infidel overthrow thy battlements. Wind and sea shall threaten your crops and the very foundations of your island. The Florentines must beware lest their lion be torn by other claws. Take care, O Venice; unexampled gales shall destroy the ships of Venice.[2]

1 Refers to the *Protestatio Bohemorum* sent by the Bohemians to the Council of Constance, 1415.　　　　　　　2 Original condensed and abridged.

Of misfortunes caused by the Conjunction some will happen only after long delay in 1563, some on the other hand come even the year before the Conjunction. Flood and shipwreck will especially be worst in February 1524. They will be worst near seas and rivers and swamplands, especially in the month of February. The *mathematicus* of Heidelberg was not alone in this forecast for 1524. Agustino Nifo of Bologna and others, though with differences, were prophesying it too. As the triennium advanced apprehension increased. In 1523 it was said[1] that men were hesitating to start new undertakings and were converting property into money as more portable.

Such astrological prognostications may be dismissed as of no account. In a sense, of course, that is so. But they are an indication of a public opinion which then existed—a 'herd-thinking' of the time. To put them aside as we do their modern successors, the 'Zadkiel' or 'Old Moore's Almanac' of to-day, is not permissible. They reflected a certain factor in contemporary opinion; they also contributed to form it. Professor Lynn Thorndike writes:[2] 'The tracts and predictions we have discussed were addressed to popes, cardinals and other prelates, to the Emperor Charles V and other secular rulers. They were composed by friars, doctors of theology, physicians and philosophers, by university professors in various fields, by historian or editor of scientific works, as well as by professional astrologers.'

The superstition they expressed, gross though it may seem, was not without influence. Astrology appealed to a wide, and in some ways cultured, audience. It was an age when the election of a Pope might be postponed until the planets were favourable. The *Practica* of Wirdung, issued in latin as well as in the vernacular, spread its net for a wide public. On the one hand, it was meant for the ear of the Church—and Luther, soon to be a power, was as superstitious as was Rome. It was to reach the lawyer and the physician. Also, as its dedication shows, it looked for a hearing from the nobility at the castle.[3] It also reckoned on the good burghers of the town, and their dames and gossips. With some it would weigh hardly less than a passage in the Apocalypse; and have the advantage of being the more *ad hoc* of the two.

1 *Libellus consolatorius*, see L. Thorndike, *History of Magic and Experimental Science*, V, 222, Tannstetter.
2 *History of Magic and Experimental Science*, v, ch. XI, p. 233.
3 Cf. T. Erastus, *De Nova Disputationum, etc.*, 4, Praefatio, Basle, 1572.

Its bias we see was toward the ruling classes. Its loyalty was to the sword; it expected things to be upset by violence and to be redressed by violence. It was in sentiment feudal. It concluded, 'may all things in heaven and earth at last revert again to the hands of a prince; Amen'. Which is Carlyle's 'O, for one hour of Duke William again', and, for that matter, at long last amounts to 'ein feste Burg ist unser Gott'.

The year 1524, when it came, proved not in fact a catastrophic one. It was a wet year in many places [1] and not without war—few years were. There was no general cataclysm of weather or war; there was a peasants' rising in Germany.

What was Fernel's reaction to this definite misadventure of astrological prediction? He was at the time reading and taking pupils as an M.A. in his own old College and University. He was, we know, sympathetic with astrology. That this misprediction did not dissuade him from astrology seems clear from the fact that less than two years later he is writing his *Monalosphaerium*, and dealing with the 'critical days'; and in the next two years there followed his two further works touching astrology and its computations—those three works on which Plancy's 'Life' remains silent.

There were astrologers who dissented from the predicted catastrophic year, many in part, a few *in toto*. Sylvestro Lucarello,[2] of Camerino, where he was professor of the 'science of the stars', writing at the end of January 1524, declared that 'the 16 conjunctions of the planets, in the sign of Pisces in the present year will not occasion either flood or drought', and he called to witness Gaurico, the astrologer, to that effect. From Gaurico himself there seems to have been no prediction for 1524 (or at least none extant), although for 1525.[3] Fernel's pursuance of astrology after the miscarriage of the prediction for 1524 may have meant that he sided with the dissentients in the controversy. He may have held that not astrology was mistaken, but only certain of its practitioners. That he was not weaned from astrology by what happened agrees well with a conclusion on the subject arrived at by Prof. L. Thorndike, summarising the whole long incident. 'Although such disagreement among the astrologers might

1 L. Thorndike, *History of Magic and Experimental Science*, v, ch. XI, pp. 231–2.
2 Prognosticon Anni MDXXIIII quo opiniones pseudo-astrologos Diluvium & Siccitatem praesentis anni falso praedicentium improbantur, etc. per Eximium Virum Syderalis Scientiae pfessorum Silvestrum Lucarellum, Camertem. Rome, the last day of January 1524. 4°.
3 L. Thorndike, *History of Magic and Experimental Science*, v, ch. XIII, p. 256.

be supposed to lessen the faith of the public in them, even the sharpest critic of others usually did not desist from predicting himself. There was no apparent let-up in the urge towards divination, and it must have catered for a correspondingly great public demand.'[1]

Fernel's own relinquishment of astrology has no appearance of being sudden. Cumulative distrust in it had deepened as his life advanced and his professional experience increased. This emancipation of himself contrasts with the fate of a copy of his *Medicina* on the bookshelves of the Duke of Saxony of that time. Part of the point and novelty of that work was, as we shall see, that it faced toward rationalism, and discountenanced astrology, and all recourse to it in medicine. Across the fly-leaf of the Ducal copy a contemporary hand (1590) has written '*fortuna potentior arte*'—the astrological motto, 'fate avails more than skill'.[2]

Plancy tells us there came a time when Fernel

condemned astrology utterly, with its genitures and divinings invented from the stars by the superstitious, and giving predictions of I-know-not-what portents and falsehoods. It fabricated a number of celestial 'houses' and 'habitations' for no other reason than to foretell favourable or adverse fortune from horoscopes, and for the imagining of a number of characters and figures from the various movements of the stars, from their 'approaches', 'aspects' and 'conjunctions'. It amounted to sheer prostitution of a pretended foreknowledge of things to come.[3]...He [Fernel] insisted that any understanding of the 'days of crisis' was in no wise to be looked for from the shallow arguments which astrology had to offer, contradicting the well-founded observations of ancient physicians, and disturbing the sequence of the decretory days. He admitted that at one time, deceived by the specious promises of astrological observation, and not yet sufficiently versed in the practice of medical art, he had thought favourably of astrology. But the really valuable thing to do was to pay attention to the onset of an illness, its progress, the nature and ways of the humours carrying it, and not least to the latent sympathy and occult harmony of the motion of the days on which these operations occur; and finally the natural strength (of the patient). By reflection on these things it might be possible to foresee and predict days, in the struggle between nature and

1 L. Thorndike, *ibid.*
2 L. Thorndike, *History of Magic and Experimental Science*, VI, 634: 'On his return to Germany [c. 1558] Erastus was shocked at the extent to which men were addicted to vain predictions of astrologers and at the astrological restrictions under which medical practice laboured.' Erastus himself was Swiss.
3 *Vita. V. infra*, bibliog. no. 68, *Appendix*, p. 197.

the disease, in which a rapid change would set in, and whether towards recovery or not, that is, with favourable or fatal issue. But the days of crisis do not result from influences of the stars and moon and their aspects, neither is dearth of the humours so brought about, nor tendency to crisis.[1]

There is nothing in Fernel's later writings to lead us to distrust this account from his faithful Plancy, written soon after Fernel's death.

But, at the time of composing the 'Dialogue', Fernel had not travelled so far in his distrust of astrology. True, in the 'Dialogue' he no longer deals with nativities and horoscopes. But he is still intrigued by astrology, and though hesitant, has not broken with it. His Preface tells how, twenty years before, he had been impressed by that sentence in Hippocrates, 'Is there not in disease something of the supernatural?' τὶ θεῖον, quid divinum? The question had become somewhat of an obsession with him. What, he asked, had been in Hippocrates' mind? The stars? Would they be truly supernatural? The 'Dialogue' has three characters, three friends. Two of them, Philiatros[2] and Brutus, meet by chance, and go to consult a third, Eudoxus, in his garden. There they put to him this question from Hippocrates. They put it to him as from themselves and as a question of to-day. Eudoxus is older than they, and a physician. In Eudoxus Fernel represents himself, taking the name of an 'astrologer' of antiquity—he styled Ptolemy 'astrologer'.[3]

Short questions notoriously may take long answers. This one does not find its answer until the tenth chapter of the second and final book. But that apart, Eudoxus is asked if living things, besides consisting of the cardinal elements, derive anything from the heavens. He replies: 'Yes; they do.' 'Equally and at all times?' asks Brutus.

---

1 *Vita. V. infra*, Note II, *Appendix*, p. 159.

2 The name Philiatros lends itself as a pseudonym to medical characters and writers; it has often been used so. An instance, in Fernel's time, is Étienne Dolet's use of it as 'éditeur' of Galen's *Therapeutics*, Lyons, 1539, 8°, Jehan Barbon. Dolet's letter on the verso of the title-page recognizes Jean Canappe as the translator, but Dolet was editor. Again, Rabelais appears to have taken 'Philiatros' as a pseudonym in translating parts of Galen's *Therapeutics*. It was the pseudonym also of Conr. Gesner. The term applied also, I think, to senior candidates for the Doctorate of Medicine at Paris, and elsewhere. Bauhin's dedication of what he entitled Fernel's 'Pharmacy' declares that it will be the more interesting to 'philiatris et pharmacopaeis' because he, Bauhin, inscribes it to the young patron he mentions. (*Pharmacia*, p. A 6. See Bibliography, *infra*, p. 205, 124.U.)

3 E.g. Consilium 53.

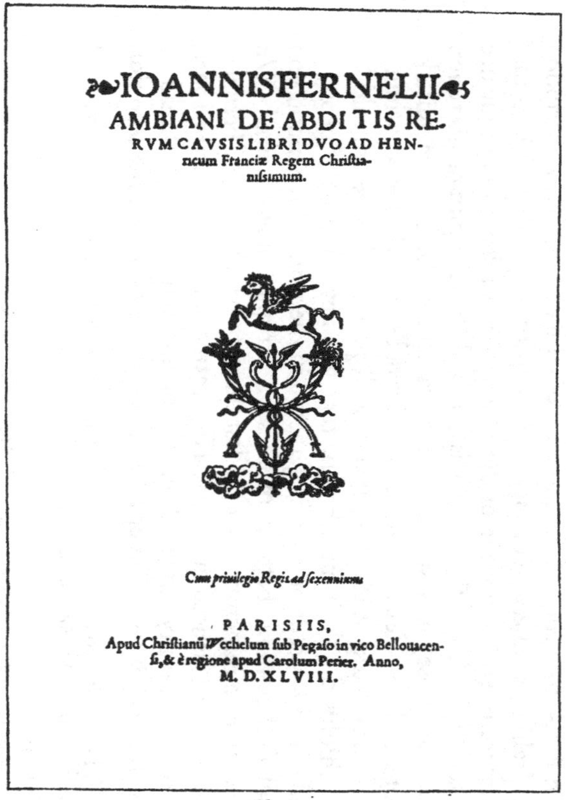

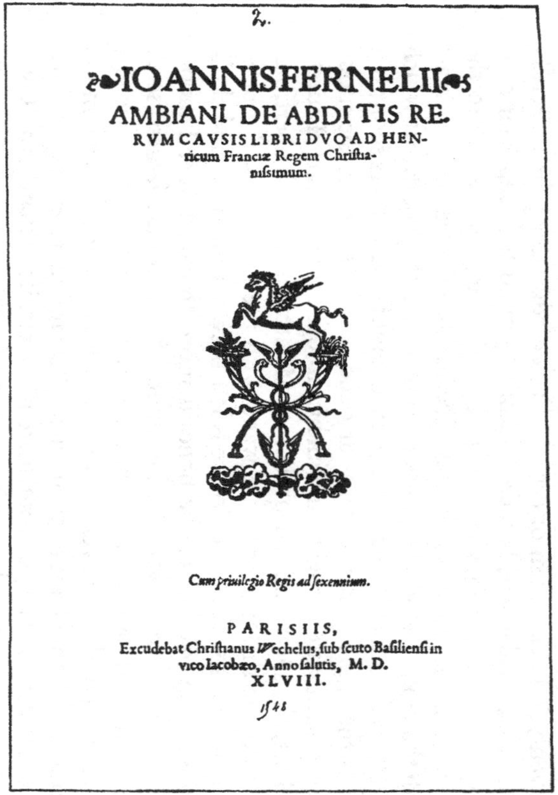

2.

IOANNISFERNELII
AMBIANI DE ABDITIS RE-
RVM CAVSIS LIBRI DVO AD HEN-
ricum Franciæ Regem Chriſtia-
niſsimum.

Cum priuilegio Regis ad ſexennium.

PARISIIS,
Excudebat Chriſtianus Wechelus, ſub ſcuto Baſilienſi in
vico Iacobæo, Anno ſalutis, M. D.
XLVIII.
1548

Fig. 8.

IOANNISFERNELII
AMBIANI DE ABDITIS RE-
RVM CAVSIS LIBRI DVO AD HEN-
ricum Franciæ Regem Chriſtia-
niſsimum.

Cum priuilegio Regis ad ſexennium.

PARISIIS,
Apud Chriſtianum Wechelum, ſub Pegaſo in vico Belloacen-
ſi, & è regione apud Carolum Periex. Anno,
M. D. XLVIII.

Fig. 7.

Figs. 7, 8. Fernel's 'Dialogue', 1548, 2°; the two variants of title-page; Christ. Wechel.

Eudoxus answers: 'No, there are gatherings of the stars when the heavenly influences sum or cancel. Each earthly thing feels specially its own particular star, because a harmony exists between their constitutions. Some things attach more to the sun, some more to the moon, some to the other planets. The shellfish on the shore increase with the moon and with the moon decrease.[1] In the woods that which is gathered under the waxing moon is moist and withers soon; but cut in the wane of the moon is dry and lasts.'[2] Even so, the moon is less potent with Fernel than with his famous contemporary, Laurent Joubert, the Dean and Chancellor of Montpellier. For Joubert, not only do the shellfish wax and wane with the moon, but the brain does so; it is for that that a space is left between the brain and skull. Likewise the marrow of the bones is more abundant at full moon, as every butcher knows. At the moon's full fruits are largest, seeds swell, the humours in the veins and spaces of the body become copious, and the cadaver decomposes more quickly. The moon dominates woman more than man. The moon rules the cardinal humour, the *pituita*, and women are more pituitous than men. Over the young the moon dominates more when new, over the old, more when old. Joubert, 'On Paralysis',[3] mentions the moon several times on a page. Even Pico, challenging astrology, admitted the 'pituitous' influence of the moon. Fernel had a famous prescription for 'falling sickness', epilepsy. 'This sickness', he wrote,[4] 'comes commonly with the wane of the moon, and is related to dominance of the pituita', in other words is cerebral, for the pituita (secretion from the nose) was supposed to come from the brain, a mistake sponsored by Vesalius' anatomy. Fernel's prescription continues: 'Take mistletoe of the oak; man's skull powdered' (we are told by Matthiolus the skull must be one that was never buried); 'peony— male peony—seeds or root (if gathered in the wane of the moon you shall find nothing better); of these 2 scruples apiece; mix.' We have here to remember that the last thing to be supposed of Fernel is that he countenanced quackery. His treatment always had its reasoned argument. To my unversed reading of this prescription, a thread of coherence in it runs: epilepsy, ailment of the brain, pituita secretion

1 Cf. H. Munro Fox, *Selene, or Sex and the Moon*, 1928 (Psyche Miniatures), and *v. infra*, Note VII, *Appendix*, p. 177.
2 *Dialog.* ii, c. 18.
3 *De paralysi quaestio ex medicina*, and *Astrologia explicata*, Lyon, 1567.
4 *Liber conciliorum*, Consil. 8; also Consil. 1.

from the brain (cold and moist); powdered skull,[1] cold and dry
(earthy) from near the brain; peony root, dry; gathered in the wane
of the moon, drier; *human* skull versus *human* brain: contraries cure.
But, of course, behind each ingredient stretched an age-long tradition,
laden with the occult. In the 'Dialogue', Brutus, in his customary
rôle of 'enfant terrible', says:[2] 'But why peony in particular? Other
herbs beside peony have the cardinal quality: dryness.' Eudoxus'
reply takes refuge in the occult. It is not an affair of cardinal qualities
purely. There is also to be remembered that which is latent in the
'total substance'. Diseases of the 'total substance' are those into
which—so the 'Dialogue' decides—the supernatural does enter, as to
which Hippocrates put his query.

Eudoxus goes on with his tale of the moon's influences. 'When
there is no moon, the ant lies still, but with the full moon runs busy.'[3]
'Selenite, the stone, retains the image of the moon even to its phases.
The magnet is in sympathy with the pole-star.'[4] 'The flowers of
chicory, and of heliotrope and scorpiurus, follow the setting sun.'[5]
'Right it is for us to scan the heavens seeking Nature's help. The
ancients did so. It is done to-day. But to-day many misuse it. To-day
some disgrace it with old-wives' superstition. Worse, some degrade
it by fraud. Some would bind the freedom of man's mind to the
fatality of the stars.'[6] That astrologers overreach and deceive is however not to say that we derive no influence from the stars. 'Who
to-day will deny that the powers of the elements and of natural
bodies are upheld and maintained by the motions and powers of the
heavens?'[7] 'Like draws like: the planets have their affinities to the
body. The temperament differs from planet to planet, as in men from
man to man, and indeed from illness to illness. This planet may help
this man in this disease and harm that man in that disease, and conversely. But when, and to what extent, and when more and when
less, or indeed if at all, that only observation can decide. We cannot

1 Jean Béguin, the pharmaceutical chemist, and author of the *Tyrocinium*, early in
the century next after Fernel, wrote of extracts of cranium as 'famous for epilepsy'.
Among remedies administered to Charles II was extract of cranium, doubtless for
his convulsions; he was dying of uraemia. (Cf. Patterson, *Annals of History of
Science*, vol. v (1937), p. 263.)

2 *Dialog.* ii, c. 17. Cf. Erastus, *Disput.* 4, p. 140.

3 *Dialog.* ii, c. 18.   4 *Ibid.* c. 17.

5 This was long an astrological argument, e.g. *Disput. d. Astrorum in Medic. Observ.
Rob. Barassin*, p. 6, Caen, 1642.

6 *Dialog.* ii, c. 18.   7 *Ibid.*

settle it in the study by mathematics. I wish, as Euripides wished, that things could converse with us, and had speech to tell us what they are.'[1]   One only of his private Consilia[2] (published after his death) mentions astrology; it gives the astrological opinion that a seventh months' child is born under Saturn—an untoward influence; but it makes no comment. It does, however, refer to Ptolemy as 'astrologer'.

There is one theme which, with Fernel, leads freely into the occult, bordering on astrology. That is the innate heat. 'Innate' heat, he says, is to be distinguished from 'elemental' heat. This latter is one of the four cardinal qualities composing the individual's temperament. But the 'innate' heat is of different origin; it enters the individual at the moment when the embryo, by the very fact of this entry, suddenly became an independent individual. Fernel's reason why this heat is not 'elemental' heat seems, at least in part, original with him. Riolan and Campolongo and Valcher refer to it as Fernel's. They[3] challenge it, along with certain other of his views, namely the relation of rheumatism to the pituitary humour, and the mode of infection of *variola*. Valcher and Campolongo defend the Arabs against

1 *Dialog.* ii, c. 18. The kindness of Professor Gilbert Murray furnishes me with the source in Euripides to which Fernel refers. It is fragment 439, quoted by Plutarch, *De Gerenda Republica* and by Stobaeus: φεῦ φεῦ, τὸ μὴ τὰ πράγματ' ἀνθρώποις ἔχειν φωνήν, ἵν' ἦσαν μηδὲν οἱ δεινοὶ λόγοι. 'Alas that things should have no voice (power of speech) to men, so that subtle words were nothing.' It is given in Nauck's *Fragmenta Tragicorum*, edit. 2, fragm. 439, p. 494 (1888). Again, attention is called to the same thought of Euripides by J. Riolan the elder. In the Preface to his commentary on Fernel's Innate Heat (*Physiol.*, bk. iv and *Dialog.* bk. ii, c. 7) he has: 'Optabat Euripides, ut vel muti essemus, vel res communi sermone nobiscum loquerentur', and Riolan dilates on this. He is addressing his father-in-law Simon Petreius, physician in Paris.

2 Consil. 53 of 1582 edition, but 55, p. 375, vol. II of the 1656 edition of collected works.

3 *De Arthritide liber unus: De Variolis alter; ex Æmilio Campolongi Medicinam Theoreticen in celeberrimo Gymnasio Patavino summa cum laude profitentis explicationibus decerpti.* Nunc primum in lucem editi Opera atque industria Ricardi Valcheri Londinensis Phil. et Med.; Venice, Paolo Meieto publisher, Padua, 4°, 1586. The first work is dedicated to 'Rever⁰ Dom., D. Ricardo Scelleio Melitensis Militiae in Anglia Praefecto: et primo ejus Regni Baroni', namely to Sir Richard Shelley, Grand Prior of the Knights of Malta in England. See Note VIII, *Appendix*, p. 178. Also J. Riolan the elder, *Ad Librum Fernelii de Spiritu et Calido innato*, 8°, Paris, 1570. Cf. however S. Paparella, *De Calido*, iii, c. 1 and ii, c. 29: 'calor, qui est in animalibus, neque igneus est, neq; ab igne originem ducit', following Fernel.

Fernel's strictures. Fernel's argument that life lives by innate heat,[1] not by elemental heat, runs briefly thus:

At death the body's heat is extinguished, and what was the living thing becomes cold. So much is plain even to sense. A touch demonstrates it. It is perhaps not so evident in plants. Yet in them also it holds. The more sentient and active the animal the more liberal its heat. Now, consider the excellence of the sun, prime prince and controller of the world, favouring and forwarding each and every life that is. Then, if that heat from without can so cherish life, is there not within all living things a heat which cherishes what they are, a heat which is even of the same nature as the sun's? Death is the extinction of this heat, which is the innate heat. The coldness of old age dominates the material heat, the elemental heat, which is of the temperament; but old age cannot, so long as there is life, overcome the innate heat itself. It is in virtue of this heat that the snake lives, although its temperament is cold. So too mandragora and the poppy and all the herbs of frigid temperament.

These were valued for relief of fever, fever being a riot of heat from the heart, not always elemental.[2] Fernel continues:

The innate heat is superior to the elemental heat. Elemental cold avails against elemental heat, but it avails nothing against this more excellent heat which is the innate heat of living things. Therefore this innate heat is not of the same nature as fire. It comes from a different source from fire. In defining death Aristotle, with the intuition of a master, said the coldness of death comes not by mere overthrow of the temperament nor by surcharge of elemental cold, but by lapse of innate heat. Innate heat is the vital heat, and, like light, it has no contrary. Darkness is but deprivation of light. Death is deprivation of innate heat. Death demonstrates that this heat is no result of a mere mixture of the elements. Death occurs and still the body retains its elements and the shape of all its parts. We recognize our friend although his life is not there. The innate heat has fled him. It is not therefore traceable to the elements. They still compose the body. Therefore the innate heat, the vital heat, must have its source elsewhere.

He goes on to say that the innate heat comes from the starry sphere [3]—of, that is to say, the Ptolemaic universe—the stars belonging to the ceiling of the eighth sphere, next outside the sphere of Saturn. Eudoxus reminds his two friends that the heavenly sphere is itself an element, and far other than the elements we know; it is the quintessence. The eighth heaven is a great reservoir of the specific 'forms'

1 *Physiol.* iv, c. 1; cf. *Dialog.* ii, c. 7.   2 *Pathol.* iv, c. 2.
3 *Dialog.* ii, c. 7; i, c. 6, 7, 8.

of life. The planet Sol, i.e. sun, is mediator between it and terrestrial life. So it is that, by way of the sun, there enters into the prenatal child, corporeally prepared, on the fortieth day or thereabouts, the innate heat and the specific 'form', in short, the soul. Not, he adds, simply the human soul, but as Aristotle points out, the soul of the particular man. It is from the stars. It is celestial. To sum up, Sol and man beget Man. '*Sol et homo generant hominem.*'[1] This is not exactly astrology; it is of the doctrine of the 'occult ray'.

What then led Fernel to reject, against the opinion of his time, astrology as an adjunct to medicine? The answer is supplied by Plancy. Fernel was an observer. Versed more than most men in the stars as data for astrology, and versed, as he became, in the signs and vicissitudes of disease, he used his own first-hand observation to check the supposed agreement between the· behaviour of the

Similaribus partibus fua eft materia 118 19
Sol aduerfis corporibus lume impartit 71 35
Sol & homo generant hominem 54.48
Sola putredo nõ præparat corpora ad pefti
lenuam 136.18

Fig. 9. 'Dialogue', 1st edition. Item from Index, 1548, and repeated until the mid-seventeenth century.

stars and the facts of the sick room. His faithful judgement kept tally of agreement and of disagreement between them. Tested in this way astrological prediction, contrary to his own earlier expectation, and contrary to the endorsement of those around him, proved to be untrue. That was the ground of his dissent from it. We do not hear him accuse it of atheism, as in the famous diatribe of Pico of Miran-dola. Fernel said simply that it does not speak truly about disease and other things, and he parted company with it. For him, with his austerity of character, and his devotion to the cause of medicine, that was enough.

We cannot suppose that this judgement, abundantly right as we now know it to be, was reached easily. Otherwise many would have reached it. Leonicenus of Padua subscribed to astrology; so too did Cardan whom Fernel met in Paris when the Milanese physician was en route for Edinburgh and London; so too did the able

1 *Dialog.* i, c. 7, p. 76 [1548], and *tabula*. This caption is omitted however from the mid-seventeenth-century (Heurne's) edition (Utrecht, 1656) onward.

Fracastor of Verona and Laurent Joubert, the great Dean of Montpellier, not to speak of Marsilio Ficino, the old Platonist of
Florence, and many another. To most of those of his time Fernel's
revolt from astrology in medicine seemed the strange blindness of a
liberal spirit to a wonderful chapter opening out before medical
science. To-day we know it was a chastening of knowledge in the
interest of truth.

There was another source of confusion besetting the earnest
physician in that age of Fernel. Nature was thought open to interference by influences from outside Nature. Nature was thought to
be tampered with not unfrequently by causes supernatural. Man's life
and Nature were believed subject to intrusions of the anomalous.
In short, the physician had to reckon with *natural magic*. The Renaissance offered him little enlightenment on this question. To magic—
'natural' magic—Fernel had never, it would seem, felt drawn as to
astrology. Perhaps it lacked interest for him, by not involving
mathematics. Natural magic, when we turn it over in the mind,
presents possibly the most direct antithesis there can be to natural
science. The two, working in the same field as they do, are active
antagonists. Each deals for the most part with what it regards as
'fact' given by perception. So far they are alike. But they are opposed
as to what each considers adequate safeguard against deception and
mistake as to 'fact'. Natural science is at pains to eschew conditions
which might influence its judgement, e.g. predispositions of expectation, emotion, faith, desire, dreaming, and so on. It values confirmation of experiences, for instance, by repetition under like conditions;
also it asks for quantitative measurement and precision. Natural
magic as a cult does not. Far from avoiding wishful thinking, its
motive often *is* wishful thinking, it demands wonder-working. Some
of these biases of judgement carried, in Fernel's time, the mantle of
high, even divine, authority. He, in his honesty and love of truth,
wrestled manfully to elicit from them the unsophisticated truth. He
dwells on magic most where it concerns the powers of remedies
used in healing. Here again we find him more concerned with it in
the 'Dialogue' than in the *Medicina* of twelve years later. Nature,
the 'Dialogue' declares, has certain secrets which she likes us to
marvel at, but not to probe. For instance, the pull of the magnet upon
iron. 'I remember to have seen selenite in a ring which on mere
contact with the bare skin arrested bleeding; worn on the third finger

in the equinox it stopped dysentery.'[1] He gives other instances. He thinks they turn essentially on 'occult affinity', or on 'occult opposition'; the terms he prefers are 'sympathy' and 'antipathy'. His tone here differs from that of the Preface to the 'Therapeutics' twelve years later, where he declares roundly there is nothing in the whole of medicine *outside* the laws of Nature.

Nevertheless, in the 'Dialogue' he is incredulous of much of the magic which for the most part his contemporaries accepted as legitimate. Cardan we know, from his own lips,[2] believed in magic; he said it had forced itself into his own life many times, and he gave instances. Our own Linacre despatched finger-rings, which had received a special blessing, to his friend Budé, the humanist, in France, to be distributed for curing rheumatism.[3] Fernel is far more critical. Though even he can speak of the 'truly magical'. He accepted Ulysses' Circe as truly a witch. An impression in the Middle Ages and Renaissance was that magic had been of more frequent occurrence in the past. Holy Writ attested to past magic. Discussing Hippocrates' query, 'Is there anything praeternatural in disease?' Eudoxus (Fernel) says:

Some disease there may well be which is praeternatural, and then the remedy must be praeternatural. The praeternatural remedy can only be divine or magical. In Holy Scripture we read of the divinely supernatural, wrought by Christ and his apostles and the prophets. The magical, on the other hand, is the work of evil men imitating, by means of demons, the divine, as when Pharaoh's magicians copied the miracles of Moses, and as when Simon Magus astonished the apostles. Pliny relates that Prince Nero had in his time learned the art.[4]

Our wise laws [says Fernel] have passed many penalties against it. No magic can create the real thing as it is; it can only produce a semblance or ghost of a thing, which deceives the mind as does a conjuror's trick. Hence magic does not cure; it is never sure or safe; it is always capricious and perilous. I have seen a jaundice of the whole body removed in a single night by a scrap of writing on a paper hung round the neck. But the malady soon returns, and may be worse than before. The cure is plainly fictitious and merely makeshift.

But, he goes on, apart from these mysteries, there are a number of empty, inept superstitions which have long played on human frailty. They include things of which no man can say why they are believed

1 *Dialog.* ii, c. 17.   2 *De Vita propria Liber*, 1575.
3 P. S. Allen, *Age of Erasmus*, p. 218.   4 *Dialog.* ii, c. 16.

or whence belief in them ever arose.[1] They derive neither from 'temperament' nor from the 'manifest qualities', nor from the 'total substance', nor from magic, nor from the divine. Of such are bits of writing, signs, ligatures, rings, and so on, which rely neither on Nature nor on God, nor on the spirit world. A scrap of writing! how can it avail against disease? In medicine every effect is traceable to contraries, contraries within the same category; being cognate up to a point, they the more perfectly oppose. How can the quality 'heat' counteract a 'sound', or a sound counteract a 'shape'? Such superstition accredits occult powers to purely natural objects irrespective of their nature.

Brutus begs for examples. Eudoxus replies:[2] it is said vomiting can be stopped by certain ceremonial words, pronounced in the sick room, or even not needing to be pronounced at all. Cato treated dislocations by means of song, and so Theophrastus sciatica. I have had a colleague whose practice was to arrest bleeding by repeating over and over 'from His side went forth blood and water'. Homer tells how Ulysses stayed the bleeding of his wound by a song. Some claim that fever can be cured by saying, over the patient's hand, 'let this fever be to thee as easy as was Christ's birth to the Virgin'. Some help childbirth by saying aloud, before each labour-pain, 'exaltabo te, Deus, meus rex.'[3] The word *abracadabra*, fairly written, is tied round the neck to relieve fever, and especially quotidian ague.[4]

Fernel is objecting to all these, not subscribing to them. His criticism of one group of them runs thus: you are, by night, to administer to a case of epilepsy spring-water in the scalp of a man killed by fire. Again, for protection against the bite of a mad dog, you are to administer a pill made from the scalp of one who has been hanged. Again, for toothache you are to scarify the painful gum with the tooth of a man killed by violence. Fernel's comment is, 'whether the tooth or the scalp derives these powers from the "temperament" or from the "total substance", the tooth or the scalp of any man soever enjoys the same powers, and the manner of his death makes no difference to that. The violent death, whether by hanging or by any other means, does not affect the "temperament" or the total substance of the tooth or scalp. Neither does human scalp or tooth provide in its "temperament" or "total substance" any "contrary" for epilepsy, or for toothache, or for rabies. The alleged cause of cure

1 *Dialog.* ii, c. 16.   2 *Ibid.*
3 Vulgate; Psalm 21, 10.   4 *Dialog.* ii, c. 16.

is therefore unreasonable.' A similar argument disposes of a host of
vaunted remedies—frog's eyes plucked out and cast into hot water
before sunrise, for tertian ague; a living spider shut in a walnut shell
and hung round the neck, for quartan ague; etc. But there were
further complications. There was the claim that a remedy obtained
from the living world might be efficient when it was alive but not
when it was dead. Fernel inclined to think that this claim might be
correct. His argument was that the curative power might be an
attribute of the 'form'—the Aristotelian 'form'—in short, of the
living remedy, but not of the dead one. It is attested, he says,[1] that
the heart of the swallow, if it is to cure loss of memory, must be
administered while still beating, and, for intermittent fever, the heart
of the pigeon while still warm. In all this Fernel, and his Renaissance,
proud as he was of it, were really in no better case than had been the
Middle Ages they so held in contempt. Fernel himself, trying to test
experience against a reasoned frame of reference, was perhaps, in that
respect, more lonely than had he lived three centuries earlier. This
scepticism of his was in fact 'natural science in the making'. By his
doubt of 'magic' he was assisting the birth of natural science.

Riolan's Commentaries on the writings of Fernel possess the more
interest because they treat their theme with considerable indepen-
dence. Judging from the dates of their issue (so far as known to me[2])
they began to appear 12 years after Fernel's death, and the last published was that on the 'Dialogue', 50 years after the 'Dialogue's' first
printed issue. They give an impression of being competitive with,
rather than purely elucidative of, the Fernel texts. The so-called
Compendium Universae Medicinae does not even mention Fernel's
name in its title. The Commentary on the 'Dialogue' does in its preface
allude briefly to Fernel and with high respect. Riolan calls him 'my
friend and fellow-countryman'—Fernel had been dead many years.
It will be remembered that fifty years later William Harvey, replying
to the criticism on the 'circulation' put forth by Riolan fils—the son
of the commentator—makes the remark to him 'your admired Fernel'.
Riolan the elder's unconstrained commentary on the 'Dialogue'
multiplies the 'Dialogue's' instances of alleged magical cures. Thus it
adds as a charm for stopping bleeding the words 'may the blood stay
in thy veins as in Christ's'. It appends to the title of Fernel's bk. ii,
c. 16, 'a full discussion of whether an amulet keeps illness away'.

1 *Dialog.* ii, c. 18.   2 Note IX, *Appendix*, p. 179.

But it endorses Fernel's warning as to the magical and what can be accepted of it and what not. Finally, Riolan says 'I count myself an Aristotelian'. 'Aristotle, this side of controversy wrote much more subtly on Nature than did Plato, and on God more divinely.' Plato he blames for inventing crowds of daemons. He says he is not one to give credence rashly, but he does believe with Galen that there are properties which are occult as well as those which are manifest. 'But I, Riolan, to this day have not seen anything supernatural; hence I pay little heed to magical results taking them to be self-deceptions or the deliberate frauds of Cacodaemon.' On Fernel a stricture that he does pass is that Fernel does not give in his writings play enough to Christian faith and morals. He remarks that even Aristotle, at his last end, cried '*Ens entium miserere me*'.[1] Whence Riolan had this is not said; it savours of the medieval.

There was in Fernel's time yet another side to the occult. Of it too he took account, interested though sceptical. This was alchemy. Erastus,[2] their contemporary, who had no use for Bombastus, the self-styled 'paracelsus', yet spoke with respect of Fernel as a chemist. But Fernel himself did not actually practise alchemy. Nor did he look with favour on the metallic remedies, that is, the alchemical. He had seen the harm done by quicksilver in the new disease, the *lues venerea*, now called syphilis. It was, however, not the quicksilver but its over-dosage which in fact was wrong. Our point here is that though, as Thevet says, Fernel condemned 'paracelsing',[3] yet on behalf of medicine, he kept track of what alchemy was doing.

Alchemy had been busy for centuries, in Christendom and in Islam, and indeed before Christendom or Islam were. The alchemist believed, as did many, that Nature consisted of more than met the eye; but, unlike others, he was not content to sit and look on; he tried to pry out by way of experiment. He actively tested Nature. His aim may have been chiefly to find the road to wealth; with some, that may have been their sole impulse, but, at least, they sought to make use of Nature by understanding her. They attempted to wrest her secrets from her by opening her hand. They subjected her substance to repeated experiment, analytic and synthetic. In

1 *Comment. de abd. rer. Caus.* p. 32, Paris, 1598.
2 Erastus (Thom.), *Disputationum partes*, IV, Basle, 1572.
3 *Les Vrais Pourtraits des Hommes Illustres*, bk. VI, p. 568, Paris, 1584.

this they were pursuing a plan which others neglected. But they obstructed their own progress by a habit of jealous secrecy. Each alchemist kept closely to himself his knowledge and his findings. He was a slave to 'growing gold', and worse, to growing gold for himself. He was, too, in several ways, of tainted repute. A discipline steeped in the occult Fernel could have condoned; he admitted the occult, if to his judgement well attested. Fernel's quarrel with the alchemist was that same which had been Geoffrey Chaucer's two centuries before—its lapse from honesty. Fernel says, though I cannot now find the place, 'when a man has the truth, it should be in some sort a point of honour with him to bear witness to it'. Furtiveness clung to alchemy. It thus sinned against the open altruism of the true scientific spirit. A precept of science is free interchange of scientific knowledge. 'Science', said Rutherford in one of his last lectures, 'goes step by step and every man depends on the work of his predecessors. It is mutual influence which makes the enormous possibility of scientific advance. The combined wisdom of thousands of men, all thinking about the same problem.'[1] The alchemist concealed from others such knowledge as he thought he had. The routine of alchemy devised secretive systems by which to hide what it did, and what it saw. It invented cryptic alphabets and cyphers for that purpose. Allegory became with the alchemist a habit of mind. Part of the obscurity and equivocality which infests Bombastus,[2] may, if we are charitable, be plausibly ascribed to this. Anagrams and acrostics masked the alchemist's 'results'. His apparatus and steps of procedure were indicated by symbols taken

1 *Background to Modern Science*, edited by Needham and Pagel, p. 73, 1938, Camb. Univ. Press.

2 *The Way to Succeed* (edit. princeps, 1612), after some passages in imitation of 'Paracelsus' (cap. 35), adds, 'it was all as plain as a nightingale crying mustard in the street'; Stonor's translation, vol. 1, London, 1930. Arpe's *Theatrum Fati* remarks, 'tam obscura proponeret dogmata ut Paracelsus, si reviveret, Paracelsum vix intelligeret'. Again, regarding the same character, Fernel's genial colleague, Jean Riolan père, later Dean of Medicine in Paris, after exposing his shams in various ways, wrote: 'Sed cur laboro in eo refellendo, quem omnes Academiae ut hominem...capitalem hostem veritatis...exegerunt?' (*Joan. Riolani in libros Fernelii...commentarii*, p. 202, 8°, Mompelgarti (Montbeliard), Jacob. Foyllet, 1588). Generosity, however, asks some allowance for this strange figure. An 'inferiority complex' attaching to concealed physical defect might explain his habitual arrogance and trickery. No servant was loyal to him. The portrait in the Louvre (by van Schoorl) is of markedly feminine appearance. For a documented account of him, see R. A. Liénard's *Paracelsus*, 8°, Paris, 1932.

from the names of plants and animals. Even for these he avoided
taking any common basis, lest their privacy be lost. These conceal-
ments were of a piece with his main interest—getting gold. Alchemists
had gold-fever as badly as any nineteenth-century mining camp.
Alchemy, looked back at, was a veiled figure, whispering secrets
which were, in fact, illusory. One of its secrets was the 'philosopher's
stone'.

There were the metals. Seven, like the planets—seven pervaded
the occult. Of the seven metals five—quicksilver, copper, iron, tin
and lead—were 'base', two—silver and gold (moon and sun)—were
'noble'. The metals sprang from seed, and Nature transmuted seeds.
For instance, the cardinal elements; each of the cardinal elements
presented a conjunction of two of the four elemental qualities. Thus,
water, the cardinal element, combined elemental moisture and
elemental cold. Treated with heat its elemental cold was displaced
by elemental heat; water, the element, was thus transmuted to
elemental air (vapour), a conjunction of elemental wet and elemental
heat. This transmutation was plain for all to read, and Nature commonly performed it, as also a number of others not unlike it. Man
could also perform transmutations. Thus, there was one with galena.
Differing from lead, it is not to be melted and is not malleable, but
it has the tint and sheen of lead. Heated, it gives off fumes of sulphur
and is transmuted to lead. It was inferred—and thought obvious—
that, if from that lead more sulphur were expelled, there would result
the nobler metal silver, and ultimately, from that, the still nobler gold.

Nature was constantly engaged in transmutations. Nature produced wheat and flowers from earth and rain. Animal growth itself
was a kind of transmutation. Lucretius in some well-known lines
sang that the wheat's meal became flesh. Within the earth Nature
produced silver and gold, transmuting the base metals into them.
Nature had powers at command, and lengths of time at command,
beyond those available to man. Tradition, however, averred that
there was a substance, a preparation, which could be produced, and
had been produced, by wise men, with special power to transmute
the base metals into gold. This preparation was known as the 'elixir'
or 'philosopher's stone'. Certain alchemists in past ages had possessed
this secret. The old Hermetic scripts contained it written in cryptic
terms—the scripts of Hermes Trismegistus. And Hermes Trismegistus? 'At the time when Moses was born, there flourished Atlas
the astrologer, brother of Prometheus Physicus, and grandfather, on

the mother's side, of the elder Mercurius, whose nephew was Hermes Trismegistus'; so the neo-Platonist Marsilio Ficino of Florence, introducing to Cosmo de Medici his translation of the *Power and Wisdom of God*.[1] Hermes Trismegistus had had the secret of breeding gold and had written it down. And after him others had done so. In fourteenth-century Paris there had been Nicolas Flamel, 'le faiseur d'or', who had a MS. from Abraham the Jew.[2] It was a recipe for 'growing gold'. Receipts, purporting to be the original, were still bruited about, darkly. The story still circulated in Fernel's time, that Raymond Lulle had come to London to grow gold for King Edward III, whence that fine gold piece, the 'rose noble'. A statute of 5 Henry IV made it felony 'to multiply gold or silver or to use the art of multiplication'. This is perhaps a context to the growth of Shylock's ducats. Alchemy hugged to itself this tradition of 'multiplying' gold. The 'elixir' or 'philosopher's stone' turned on it; it was a ferment for producing gold—also, as was often said, for lengthening life.

Fernel, physician, faced by problems of nutrition and growth, and by the resemblance of the great second coction, the source of the blood, to wine-fermentation, could not but be interested in alchemy's 'fermenting' of gold. What was his reaction to it? The 'Dialogue' supplies an answer. Fernel chooses the character Brutus to set forth the claims of the 'philosopher's stone'. Brutus, we saw, was not a physician but a layman of liberal view and culture: Brutus can quote[3] appositely from Augurello. Fernel opens the theme of the 'philosopher's stone' by putting into the mouth of Brutus a couple of lines of verse, and announcing them as Augurello's. This would whet the reader's palate for what was to follow. The great public of the time had actively taken sides on the question of the 'philosopher's stone'. Giovanni Aurelio, of the noble family of Augurello, from Rimini, had, despite years and failing sight, indited to Pope Leo X a poem on the subject of the making of gold—nearly 2000 hexameters. Giovanni was a genial humanist, widely popular, and, in his turn, a devoted admirer of many humanist friends, Bembo, Ficino, Politian, Aldo Manutio, Hermolaus Barbarus and others. His poem had been something of a best seller. First published at Venice (Simon de

1 Paris, 1494, Wolfgang Hopyl, rue St Jacques, at the sign of St George, small 4°.
2 Cf. Albert Poisson, *Histoire de l'Alchimie*, 8°, Paris, 1893. Flamel was an official scribe of the University.
3 *Dialog.* ii, c. 18.

Luere) in 1515 it ran to, besides further editions, three translations into french. Its author was looked upon as a scientist, as well as poet and scholar. He was of Ficino's Platonist Academy in Florence. He had many followers, and it came as a disappointment to him when, on Giorgio Valla's Chair falling vacant, Sabellico and not himself succeeded to it. A circle of friends surrounded him in his retirement at Treviso. When his mule one afternoon strayed with him, small in frame and advanced in years, into the river, the villagers braved danger to fetch him out.

He had begun his alchemical poem, *Chrysopoeia*, at the incoming of the new century; he must have been seventy years old when it first saw light from the press. It then, however, reached a public already agog with the *pros* and *cons* of its theme, alchemical gold-making. Brutus is a believer in the powers of the 'philosopher's stone'. He expatiates on it to the scholarly young Philiatros and the mature Eudoxus (Fernel). He mentions[1] a quintessence with occult powers, which he describes as, finally, more pure than is the purest blood. It is purified by successive refinings, reminding us of Fernel's account of the work of the brain, where by a suite of refinings the crude Galenical spirit of the senses is gradually freed from all corporeal dross and converted into the utterly pure spiritual substance of the intellect.[2] Brutus, continuing about his quintessence, says of it that, seven times distilled, it is eventually shaken in a narrow-necked flask and driven up and down until finally hardly a trace of impurity remains. He concludes, 'It is effective of much'.

Philiatros exclaims: 'You bring us a great deal of the abstruse. I wager you can tell us stranger things yet. Perhaps you are on the track of the famous philosopher's stone.' Brutus replies: 'On the track? No; say rather already arrived.' Then Philiatros: 'Perhaps to your great loss.' Brutus answers: 'On the contrary, to my great gain and encouragement. What you dismiss as fable and fiction, is a splendid asset and prize.' Philiatros: 'What is it, I ask.' Brutus rejoins: 'It were wrong to impart this thing to the profane.' Here Eudoxus interposes: 'The day draws late. Brutus, do as you are asked. Friends have no secrets one from another as to what each accepts in his philosophy.' Brutus concedes: 'At your request, I will speak. Not that I shall set forth the treasure in all its fullness; I shall declare simply that of which I have actually first-hand knowledge.

1 *Dialog.* ii, c. 18.   2 *Physiol.* vi, c. 10, and c. 14.

Lest however your unfamiliarity with terms and phrases, which our forefathers used as a precaution to hide their discoveries, make the truth difficult for you, I will reveal it frankly in the plainest words. Yet only in outline, and as briefly as I may. Know then that the "philosopher's stone", the elixir of the Arabs, the true seed whence to generate and grow gold, is not to be sought in or traced to sulphur or quicksilver, or to any of the many other things so often alleged. It is to be found solely in gold and in gold of the purest.' At this point he again cites—though not by name—the alchemist[1] poet Augurello—to the effect that just as the seeds of barley are in barley so 'the seeds of gold are in gold'.[2]

With that as a text he then enters on the recital of a long and complicated alchemical recipe for turning a smaller quantity of gold into a larger quantity. The procedure includes resort to an excerpt, engraved on an amethystine tablet, from a script of Hermes Trismegistus. The end-result is that this true elixir and ferment, acting on the fertile seed of gold, produces from one drachm of gold two hundred and fifty. Poured into two hundred and fifty of fluid lead or tin it will convert the whole mixture into gold of the purest quality. 'An immense treasure', cries Brutus exultingly. 'As the poet sang, "let but a tiny piece be cast upon the waves of ocean, and if that ocean be quicksilver the whole expanse from shore to shore

1 Joannes Aurelius Augurellus (1441–1524), canon of Treviso, author of *Carmina*, 1491, Verona, 4°, *Chrysopoeia and Geronticon*, 1515, Venice, 4°.
2 The lines given in Fernel's 'Dialogue', p. 247 (edition 1548), run:

Hordea cui cordi, demum serit hordea, ne tu
Nunc aliunde pares auri primordia: in auro
Semina sunt auri, quamvis abstrusa recedant
Longius, et multo nobis quaerenda labore!

They are from the *Chrysopoeia*, book i, 1515 edition. In the vernacular edition of Fernel's time they were rendered:

Pour cueillir l'Orge il fault l'Orge semer
Donques affin qu'en peine Coustumiere
De l'Or la source et semence premiere
Ne soit par toy cherchee vainement
Ce poinct tu doibs croire certainement
Qu'enclose en l'Or de l'Or est la semence.
Combien qu'avec grand peine et diligence
Ceste semence en ses secrets cachee
S'acquiert par nous quand elle est bien cherchee.

Fol. 24 recto, '*L'Art de faire l'Or*, traduict par F. Habert de Berry', Paris, 1550, dedicated 'à très noble, et scientifique personne, Monseigneur Pierre d'Acigné, Chanoine et Thresorier de Nantes'.

will be converted into pure gold"!'[1] 'Ah, ah,' says Philiatros, 'what is this I hear! I devote all I possess to the prosecution of this astounding adventure!' But Eudoxus intervenes. He rebukes Brutus. 'How can you so prostitute philosophy to lucre; it is as though you lust after gold. Can you not perceive how utterly fabulous is that last statement of yours? Let us put it aside, that ridiculous story about treasure. Let us, instead, extract, from what you have told us, what there is of genuine, what of so to say pure, in this great field of the occult. Brutus, for having clearly disclosed to us what you have, accept our best thanks.' Brutus rejoins: 'On my part I can never thank you enough for all I owe you.' We can infer that Fernel, while rejecting the 'philosopher's stone' as fable, thought it yet worth while to hear about it, for light which it might throw on the occult. And this attitude is entirely in harmony with him throughout the 'Dialogue'.

Looking back we know now that alchemy, by its experiments, was in course of time to found a new system of knowledge, which, from its long apprenticeship to alchemy, would be called, at first a little slightingly, chemistry. But Fernel was of the Renaissance, and the Renaissance did not come into that story. The new knowledge, Chemistry, when later it came, would create a new Medicine—the Medicine of to-day—because the body and its ways would be found to be in the main chemical. This new Medicine and its chemistry would be a part and parcel of science in general, and Medicine would become merged in the broad stream of science. But the Renaissance did not glimpse that. Nor was it given to Fernel to foresee this development from alchemy. To no one of his time was it given. Yet 'Magic is the lineal ancestor of modern science' (Sir W. Dampier).

As for that question from Hippocrates, which started the 'Dialogue', 'Is there anything supernatural in disease?' what is the 'Dialogue's'

---

1 The lines in Fernel's text, p. 249, are:

> Ipsius ut tenui projecta parte per undas
> Æquoris, argentum si vivum tum foret aequor,
> Omne vel immensum verti mare posset in aurum.

They are book iii, *Chrysopoeia* (fol. kii verso). The Paris vernacular version renders them:

> Que si en Mer tu viens un peu jecter
> De ceste pouldre acquise par art gent
> Et que la Mer fust lors tout vif Argent
> Par ceste pouldre et petite partie
> La Mer seroit toute en Or convertie.

answer to it? It is reached late (bk. ii, c. 10). It is supplied by Eudoxus. It runs thus. Disease is for the most part natural, a disturbance of the temperament, of the balance of the four cardinal qualities. But, over and above natural disease, there are certain diseases of another kind, corruptions of the total substance (*tota substantia*). Now the nature of total substance is, Eudoxus admits, difficult to expound. Total substance is akin to Aristotelian 'form'. Its corruption is not a putrefaction; it is rather an exhaustion of the innate heat.[1] There is therefore disease which directly attacks the heaven-sent 'form', or total life, as such. Eudoxus is asked what support he finds in Galen for this. He replies that Galen, when dealing specifically with this question put by Hippocrates, did not go beyond referring to an evil principle in the air. But Eudoxus cites then another passage from Galen, which calls to witness the 'total substance' and its vulnerability. His hearers are satisfied by that. There are diseases of the 'total substance'.[2] What diseases are they? Eudoxus goes on. They are plague and pestilence. They spread by invisible means, unseeable seeds. They are diseases which go by various names. They have, however, one feature in common, namely that their immediate cause is always utterly unknown, is, in short, beyond our sense—in a word, occult. That is what Hippocrates was meaning. That is the answer reached by the 'Dialogue' to the question it set out with.

The 'Dialogue'[3] is a very human document. It takes us into its confidence on a number of vexed questions. It is intimate enough with us to make us wonder what exactly were the hesitations its author had about its publication. We know Fernel was to change his mind about some of its questions. In his latest work, the still unfinished 'System of Medicine' of four years before his death, he would, as already said, declare that the whole book of healing was nothing other than a copy of the code of inviolable laws observable in Nature. Then, at last, he was to have no exceptions to the operation of Natural Law, apart only from the Human Reason and Human Free-Will. In

1 Cf. *supra*, p. 39.
2 Erastus, T., *Epistle to Crato*, Sept. 1575, attacks this. Tiguri, 1595.
3 The 'Dialogue' was first printed by Christian Wechel of Paris (1485–1554), founder of the firm, and of Flemish origin. He was one of 'the 24 printers of Paris'. He was famous as a printer of Greek and his Greek type is found in the 'Dialogue'. He printed for Erasmus and for Rabelais. Bibliog. 17.F1.

effect, Fernel was among the relatively few, who, as they enter advanced years, grow more modern.

The 'Dialogue' secured a wide audience early, and it retained readers for several generations. There were issues of it in Venice, Lyons and Geneva as well as Paris. It was printed more than thirty times within a century. It and its author were sufficiently familiar to the public to be pilloried by name in that pseudo-Rabelaisian medley, the *Moyen de Parvenir*.[1] There[2] Gorreus is made to tease Fernel with having confused 'effects' with 'causes' in his 'Dialogue'— Gorreus being Jean de Gorris, Dean of the Paris Faculty in the year when the 'Dialogue' was first printed. All of which goes to indicate that the 'Dialogue's' public was not confined to purely medical circles.

The fame and practice of Fernel increased. He addressed the Preface of his 'Dialogue' to the king, namely to that same prince to whom, as dauphin, he dedicated his treatise on 'The Natural Part of Medicine' (1542). A straightforward unembroidered dedication, presupposing on the part of the prince an active interest in, and at least a conversational familiarity with, medicine, its theory and practice. Fernel was knit to Henri II by several ties; one was the 'saving the life' (1543) of Mistress Diane de Poitiers, later Duchess of Valentinois. With Henri's accession to the throne, at the death of Francis I, Fernel could have become at once physician-in-chief to the king. With all duty, however, he begged himself off. Plancy's 'Life' recounts the incident. Fernel pleaded 'ill-health', but a more sincere plea would have been reluctance to leave Paris, his students, and his practice, for Fontainebleau. His pupils were carrying his fame

1 By Beroalde de Verville.

2 *Moyen de Parvenir*, chap. 25: '*Gorreus*. Truly, brother, this story of yours has made me laugh so much that I've done some intellectual lantern-work of my own, similar to our friend's above; so you can believe that I laugh with a lighter liver.

'*Fernel*. Why liver?

'*Gorreus*. Because according to the teaching of your book *De abditis Rerum Causis*, which should rather be *Effectis*, since you don't deal with causes but only with effects, we are to regard as the source of pleasure this fine liver-wind which wafts unseen about our insides exciting joyful melodies when mirth or dinner is desiderated.'

(*The Way to Succeed*, by Beroalde de Verville, newly done into English by Oliver Stonor. The Hesperides Press, MCMXXX.)

Jean de Gorris published (Paris, 1564) *Definitionum medicarum*, lib. xxiv; also edited Hippocrates, etc.

over Europe, and his writings were being printed in Lyons and Venice as well as in Paris. Fernel had in effect said to the king: 'Master de Bourges [1] was physician to your father. Retain him and let me wait.' King Henri had granted the request, but unwillingly. He looked on

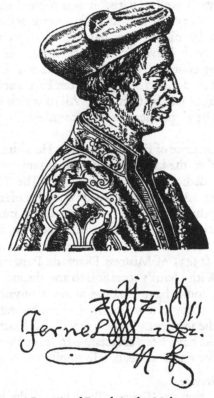

Fig. 10. Portrait of Fernel, in the *Medicina*, 1554.

Fernel as the guardian of his health. Not that Henri was cowardly about illness. He was to die, and die gallantly, of a hideous tourney wound,[2] after some days of lingering. Master Ambroise Paré, the

1 Louis de Bourges became chief physician to King Francis I in 1525. Born in 1482, and christened, it was said, under the auspices of Louis of Orleans, he was admitted doctor at the age of twenty-two, out of regard to his father Jean, then the 'father' of the Paris Faculty. Retained, at the instance of Fernel, in the post of first physician of the king, under Henri II, he died in December 1556. Fernel then succeeded him. Louis de Bourges had been with Francis at the battle of Pavia.

2 Note X, *v. infra, Appendix*, p. 180.

surgeon, would be there, and the emperor's physician, Vesal, but not Fernel. The trusted physician would himself have passed away a year before the king.

If we ask what he was like in form and features—this man, whose words we have been reading—the *Medicina* of 1554, from Wechel's press, has a woodcut which seems the only contemporary portrait. For the printed book to give a portrait of the author had become not unusual by the mid-sixteenth century, especially with issues of classical and patristic writers. Sometimes the same figure did duty for more than one author. Ovid on this occasion, Livy on that. Later, portraits of living authors were supplied in their works. An instance is that of Savonarola, in his tracts by Miscomini in Florence, 1495–6. In Fernel's time to give such portraits was fairly common. Ambroise Paré, Guillemeau, Laurent Joubert, Cardan, are instances. The woodcut of Fernel was rather earlier than these. It was reproduced by the Wechel firm many times in succeeding editions. That it was reproduced often in its own day suggests that it had some fidelity.

For other portraits of Fernel a list in Note XI gives such as I have met with. Further, a window in the Cathedral of Beauvais contains a St Luke which is credited with being a portrait of Fernel.[1] In 1794, the young French Republic—in its year III—when seeking to put an end to the old breach which had in France separated medicine and surgery for many successive centuries, created the comprehensive title 'Officier de Santé' to cover both physician and surgeon under one term. A medal was then used to commemorate 'La Médecine rendue à son unité primitive'. The obverse gives the portraits of Fernel and Paré, in profile, that of Fernel the nearer (fig. 11 frontispiece). It is evidently after the woodcut of 1554. The commemoration would seem to be mindful of the liberal[2] attitude Fernel had taken in his time, in the long feud which the young Republic sought to end. The Academy of Surgery at its foundation had, we may suppose, chosen the portraits of Fernel and Paré for its medal, as symbols of the unity of Surgery with Medicine which a reactionary past had so often in effect denied.

Regarding this medal portrait, Dr La Chronique, in his *Historical*

1 Dr P.-A. Capitaine, in his Dissertation for the Med. Facult. Paris, in 1925, wrote: 'On entering the Salle des Pas-Perdus of the Faculty, the first bust on the left is that of Fernel': *Un grand Médecin du XVIe Siècle, Jean Fernel*, Paris, 1925, 8°.

2 'Pathology', Preface to book vi.

Study of the Medals and Tokens of the Académie Royale de Chirurgie 1731–1793, states:

The final meeting of the Academy of Surgery took place on 22 August 1793, and its minutes record that the Academy, in obedience to the law (in the form of the decree by the Convention, 8 August 1793—at the height of the Terror—, which suppressed by implication all scientific associations, and confiscated their property, including the prizes 'called perpetual'), resolved that 'the meeting is dissolved'.

The conflict between physicians and surgeons thus found itself terminated. The Convention had brought all together. One thing remained over: the die which had served for striking the medal commemorating the erection of the School of Surgery. When the decree of the 14th frimaire, year III (4 December 1794) organized the 'Écoles de Santé', and installed that of Paris in the building which had been the Academy, a medal was struck carrying on its obverse the images, side by side, of Jean Fernel and Ambroise Paré, and its reverse carrying *in exergue* the legend 'Regia Munificentia'. These words disappeared only after a discussion in the École de Santé, 19th brumaire, year VI, held regarding practical instruction in the School; it was then decided to have a medal for award as a prize. The size of the medal was fixed at first for 41 mm.; but it was actually executed of the size of 59 mm., bearing the portraits of J. Fernel and A. Paré. The reverse bore then simply the staff of Esculapius in the field with the legend 'Prize of the practical School, year VI', as described in the catalogue of Coins, No. 45 (République). 1892.[1]

The medal figured here belongs therefore to the three years' interim 1793–6, and its purpose was to commemorate the settlement of the ancient conflict between the physicians and the surgeons in Paris and France. The infant Republic saw in Fernel, along with Ambroise Paré, a symbol of the reconciliation.

Fernel had dwelling with him for ten years his younger friend and assistant, the humanist physician, Guillaume Plancy. Plancy tells us something of how Fernel lived. Plancy had been a favourite pupil of the great humanist Budé, and had been entrusted with editing Budé's *Greek Epistles*. He was, we may suppose, more accomplished as a scholar than was Fernel. Lamy, writing in Paris in 1577, a few years after Plancy's death, says of him 'accomplished in Greek and Latin'. Plancy, describing Fernel's appearance, says he was tall, dark, and

1 I return here my thanks to M. Laignel-Lavastine of Paris for supplying information as to the above and other sources for the history of the medal.

strongly built. The contemporary woodcut at the age of fifty-seven shows clean-shaven lips, closed and muscular, suggesting firmness and mobility. The head is covered with the four-cornered doctor's cap. The physician of that period seems to have remained covered even in the sick room, judging from contemporary pictures. Plancy goes on to say of him that he was quick in thought and act, but always self-controlled. His face, habitually grave, and even severe, would 'when he foresaw recovery of the patient light up, and the very accent of his voice soften, in announcing the good news'.

John de Mirfeld's *Florarium Bartholomei*,[1] of the fourteenth century, has a chapter devoted to the manner and conduct called for in a physician. John de Mirfeld, a priest without benefice who lived in the Priory of St Bartholomew in London, twin foundation with the great hospital of that name, was perhaps a chaplain to the hospital. He wrote a summary of the relations obtaining, under Canon Law, between the physician and the priest attending the sick. He gives the injunction that the physician, however desperate the case, must hold out hope of recovery to the patient. He might however impart the truth to the patient's friends, if to do so seemed to him best. This rule is traceable back at least as far as the eleventh century; it is found in a 'Visit of the Physician to the Patient' by Archimatthaeus the Salernitan.[2] Plancy, describing Fernel's ways and custom in the sick room, relates this same course as his invariable practice. Convention —or more than a convention, since it was a statutory injunction of Church Law—was therefore still being preserved, after a run of six centuries. Fernel inspired confidence. Henri II of France is reported as saying, so long as he had Fernel beside him, illness would not be mortal.

With the Faculty in Paris Fernel was unpopular, but he was popular with the people. It was common knowledge that, in his busy practice, the poor received attention along with the rich. Dissent from other physicians he often did, but he was never known to speak slightingly of a professional colleague. Not that he always suffered fools gladly. A letter, answering a learned correspondent, opens: 'Not merely perfunctorily but very diligently have I read your letter through; in it there is much which is obscure, and not every disease of the joints is gout.' That Fernel had humour appears too from a

1 *Johannes de Mirfeld of St Bartholomew's, Smithfield, his Life and Works*, by Sir P. Horton-Smith Hartley and H. R. Aldridge, 1936, Camb. Univ. Press.
2 See Hartley and Aldridge above.

comment in his consultation book: 'T...... W......, a senator of B......, aged thirty-four only, but has a protruding abdominal vastness like a burgomaster's.'

Plancy records that Fernel liked, when called to a man of parts, after the diagnosis and treatment were settled, and if the state of the case and his own time permitted, to get some talk with his patient. With a philosopher on philosophy, with a geometer on mathematics, with a soldier on cities and their sites, or on engines of war and their inventors, with mariners on navigation and new countries, with divines on spirits and on God, with merchants on methods of commerce. In these talks he would contrive some point of encouragement or comfort for each patient, and would relieve a grave theme with a quiet jest or 'touch of humour'. He won affection as well as respect. In the little volume of excerpts from his consultation book, published by a pupil years after his death, a note on a young man runs: 'Sadness and fears, arising without occasion, trouble him often. He suffers from a sense of loneliness; sombre meditation thrusts itself upon him, and at night his sleep is troubled and molested by apparitions, and sundry frightments. Whence this sick gentleman, of distinguished mind and most excellent understanding, is being daunted in spirit, and is distrustful of himself, and cannot be raised to any good reliance in health.' Brief professional memorandum, this has yet a note of sympathy. Men had confidence in the character as well as in the skill of Fernel. As to the latter, Guy Patin, in one of his characteristic letters,[1] speaks of Fernel's hands as 'possessed of eyes' (*manus ocellatae*).

As to Fernel and the Faculty in Paris, Plancy's 'Life' says 'most of them hated him'. But he was too powerful to be suppressed. One source of the quarrel, Plancy says, was the attack by Fernel on the excessive blood-letting then in vogue.[2] Another, Plancy tells us, was that Fernel kept some of his prescriptions confidential to himself and a few trusted friends. He did not wish them, Plancy tells us, to be known until the book he was writing on therapeutics had been published. But, Plancy says, the hostility to him was rooted chiefly in jealousy. He gives some details about this. In his Preface to the edition of the 'Medicine' (Paris, 1567), published nine years after Fernel's death, Plancy states that the feeling against

1 To Belin, 28 October 1631.
2 This is borne witness to by Jean Riolan the younger, in a book *Curieuses Recherches sur les Escholes en Médecine de Paris et de Montpellier*, quotations from which are given by Goulin, p. 353.

Fernel in the Faculty was still bitter; and Lamy, writing from Paris ten years later, reaffirms it. Very gradually the enmity died down. Then, in 1585, we learn from Capell, an old pupil of Fernel, writing to Le Paulmier, another old pupil,[1] that Riolan (the elder) and himself, Capell, are lecturing in the Faculty on Fernel's works.[2] J. Riolan père published well-known 'Commentaries' on, and a précis of, Fernel's works in 1598, reaching another edition in 1620.[3] Even by the earlier date Fernel was already an accepted master of medicine in the Schools of Europe. This or that sentence from him would serve as a text for a lecture or as basis for a doctorate thesis.[4] Scaevola St Marthe, speaking forty years after Fernel's death, mentions that the unique compliment was paid to Fernel of having his writings set for public lectures in the Faculty during his lifetime. But that would seem a mistake, or Plancy would surely have referred to it in the 'Life'.

At last, however, even in his old Faculty, Fernel came into his due. Patin's pen was often enough dipped in gall, but never for Fernel. He wrote of him: 'He is of my Saints, along with Galen. Never prince did more for the world than our Fernel. He rescued our learning from decay and our calling from disaster. He gave the profession a new lease of life; he bequeathed it a fresh fame. I should glory more to trace descent from him than from the King of Scots or the Emperor of Constantinople.[5] It is now one hundred and two years since he died. He lies buried not far from here. I sometimes take my two sons there that they may try to be like him.'

1 Le Paulmier was one of the three witnesses to Fernel's will, executed a few days before his death.

2 *V. infra*, Bibliographical List, no. 109.R3, p. 203.

3 *Praelectiones in Libros Physiologicos et de Abditis rerum causis. Accesserunt opuscula quaedam philosophica*, Paris, 1620, H. Perier, 8°.

4 E.g. *Method. Medendi Ferneliana, enucleata & controversiarum decisionibus illustrata, necnon publico medicorum Examini subjecta a Gregorio Horstio, D. Phil. et Medico.* Wittebergae; sumptibus Bergerianis, typiis haered. Christiani Tham. 1630.

5 Cf. L. Figard, p. 52.

Part II

THE EARLIEST 'PHYSIOLOGY'

FERNEL became a great figure with the students. They found him a treasury of knowledge, and a voice with a new message. He was devoted to them; and his energy was inexhaustible. His practice grew. Plancy tells us the routine of his day. Four o'clock found him risen and in his study, to read or write until daybreak. Then he went out, to visit patients or to the Schools to lecture. Then back to his study until the midday meal, which he sometimes did not sit down to take. The meal over, he was off again, to visit the sick. At the day's end he supped with his family, and after that withdrew again to his study to read or write. He went to bed at one hour before midnight. Custom at that time began the day earlier than now. Gargantua and his tutor, we remember, started the day at four. Five o'clock seems to have been usual for commencing the University lecture day. 'We were up at 4, and, having said our prayer, went to 5 o'clock lecture, our huge [1] books tucked under one arm, writing-case and candle-stick in our hands. Lectures lasted until 10. Then, after half-an-hour for correcting our notes, we went in to dinner. From one o'clock onward we attended lectures again, and at five o'clock got back to our lodgings, went through our notes and looked up references. Supper at 6 o'clock.' Thus Henri de Mesmes, a young student at Toulouse, describes his University day there, in the year 1545.[2] An éloge pronounced over Fernel by his young com-memorator, Scaevola Ste Marthe, states that he lived habitually a nineteen-hour day. To warnings against over-taxing himself he would reply, 'Fate will give us long enough repose', quoting—true child of the Renaissance—a line from Ovid's *Amores*.[3]

After the 'Dialogue' Fernel began writing his first purely medical treatise. He entitled it 'On the Natural Part of Medicine'. A few

1 It is a law student speaking, and law books retained their folio size and gothic script long into the sixteenth century.
2 E. Frémy, *Mémoires inédits de H. de Mesmes*, 1896; quoted by A. Tilley, *Literature of the French Renaissance*, vol. 1, 1904.
3 *Amores*, II, 9, 39. The identification of this source I owe to the kindness of Mr Henry Deas, Gonville and Caius College.

years later he called it 'Physiology', a study of which he says[1] Aristotle was the founder. The earlier title was traceable to the Faculty's usage which distinguished in its studies 'things natural, things non-natural, and things contra-natural'. The healthy body

Ioannis Fernelij Ambianatis,

De naturali parte medicinæ Libri feptem, ad Henricum Francifci Galliæ Regis filiumi

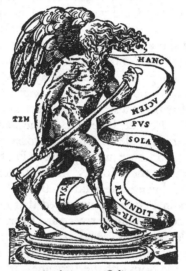

℀ Apud Simonem Colinæum;

Parifijs.
Anno M. D. XLII.
Cum priuilegio.

Fig. 12. Fernel's *De Naturali Parte Medicinae*, Paris, 1542, the de Colines' emblem said to be by Geoffroi Tory.

belonged to 'things natural', that is, which constitute our nature. Fernel's book deals with the body's healthy functioning, as then understood. It set forth the theory of the healthy body and mind, as introductory to medicine. It was issued in 1542 by Simon de Colines, as had been his earlier books on mathematics and geodesy. Its format was folio. It is, in its way, an example of first-class printer's

1 *De naturali parte Medicinae*, bk. ii, praefatio. Note XIII, *Appendix*, p. 182.

art. The two great centres of that art in France were then Paris and Lyons. The printers of Paris clustered about the old rue St Jacques, in the University quarter below Ste Geneviève. The streets around and between the Colleges had become a hive of printing and publishing. At the Sorbonne itself—the theological hub of the quarter—printing had been started some seventy years before, to promote humanism, but had, in that respect, proved premature. Those first pioneer printers had then removed to the rue St Jacques. The old historic highway ran north–south, crossing the river at the Petit Pont, next above the Pont St Michel. Civilization had footed it in shoe and sandal for perhaps a thousand years. Before housing printers, it had housed lay scribes, now displaced by the printing-presses. Even in Fernel's own day there might be met there heads grown grey disputing in the School the 'entities of substance'.

Fernel's own Collège de Ste Barbe lay hardly a stone's throw distant. As he stepped the wonderful old way Fernel would pass the doors and signs of perhaps a score of printers and publishers—'Aigle d'Or', 'Éléphant', 'Écu de Bâle', 'Homme Sauvage', and others. Sympathy with a rising tide of Church reform was not rare among these printers. It was a house just opposite to Petit's, the great printer and publisher, which, the Mornay memoirs tell us, sheltered du Plessis for a night during the wild St Bartholomew's of '72. The *Mémoire* says[1] Oudin Petit was murdered that same night. Parallel with the rue St Jacques, running riverward from Ste Barbe itself, ran the rue St Jean de Beauvais. And connecting the two, crosswise, the rue St Jean de Latran. In both of them were many printers. The 'Soleil d'Or' was the house of the Estiennes, and later of Simon de Colines. A little higher up the 'Pegasus', of the Wechels. Fernel would pass them daily. The saying was that, at the Estiennes, it was not possible to obtain discretion by speaking in latin because the very service knew latin, so cosmopolitan was the company. It was there that under the direction of Simon de Colines, successor to the business on the death of Estienne père—Henri I, as he is styled—Fernel's early 'mathematical' volumes were published.

It was, however, from an address in the rue de St Marcel that Colines issued the 'Natural Part of Medicine' of 1542. Its title-page bears Colines' device, Time with a scythe and the motto *Hanc aciem*

1 P. 105 of L. Crump's translation. Pichon and Vicaire (*Documents pour servir à l'histoire, etc.*, Paris, 1895, p. 22, footnote) cannot identify which of two, or three, Oudin Petits.

sola virtus retundit. Its draughtsman was Geoffroi Tory, poet as well as craftsman. This edition, the earliest, is now rare. Goulin, Fernel's eighteenth-century bibliographer, failed to find a copy. Renouard's monograph on Simon de Colines mentions five copies, all of them in France. There are two more in Great Britain—one of them in the Hunterian Library, Glasgow University. This latter is an exceptional copy, its capitals illuminated and coloured by a contemporary hand, its binding, contemporary, bearing, gold-stamped, the initials of the dauphin, and a dolphin with the fleur-de-lys. Fernel dedicated the book to the dauphin, whose physician-in-chief he then was. The Bibliothèque Nationale contained, before the present war, the presentation copy of Fernel's *Medicina* of 1554, dedicated to the king, Henri II, as the dauphin had by then become. The Glasgow volume may be similarly a presentation copy from Fernel himself.[1]

Of the seven books, into which the 'Natural Part of Medicine' is divided, the first (twenty chapters long) deals with human anatomy—of course merely gross anatomy, there being then no other. Begun by 1538 it pre-dates Vesalius' *De Fabrica* by a little. It is a treatise of some ninety folio pages; it is no mere compendium of the work of others. Fernel was an anatomist at first hand. He notes, for instance, that the spinal cord is hollow, 'medulla spinalis cava est',[2] which is, I fancy, the first statement of this fact. It is sometimes said (e.g. Wickersheimer[3]) to have been first described by Charles Estienne, but his volume appeared three years later than this of Fernel. The central spinal canal is a feature which escaped Vesalius altogether. An attack made, late in the eighteenth century, on Fernel's treatise on anatomy (*Histoire de l'Anatomie*, Paris, tome I) rested, Goulin shows (pp. 362–3), on mistranslations of the latin text.

Perhaps we tend to underestimate the attention given to human anatomy before Vesalius. We have to remember that in the fourteenth century Guy de Chauliac tells (1363) how his teacher Bertrucci used to proceed in dissection of the body by four stages, taking first the viscera[4] because they decayed earlier, and concluding with the limbs because they lasted longer. Guy also went on to advise what

1 The William Hunter Collection has a volume whose binding carries the combined monogram of Diane de Poitiers and Henri—the *Aulus Gellius* printed by Jenson of Venice in 1472.

2 *Physiol.* vi, c. 13.

3 *Les Médecins en France à l'époque de la Renaissance*, 8°, Paris, 1906.

4 For Fabricius' procedure cf. Howard B. Adelmann's *Fabricius*, Cornell, 1942.

sort of a body is to be chosen, much as does Fernel. In a long, special chapter Fernel gives the technical procedures of an anatomy.[1]

Fernel's 'Anatomy' is exceptional among anatomical treatises of the time—already, Fernel said, 'too numerous'—in being unillustrated by figures. The reason for this can hardly have been avoidance of expense or lack of technique on the part of de Colines' press, for the volume is, in its way, lavishly produced, and de Colines' press was equal to producing anatomical figures of the finest kind, witness not a few in Charles Estienne's *De Dissectione* equal in design to Vesalius' *De Fabrica* (by Oporinus of Basle).[2] The absence of 'pictures' from Fernel's 'Anatomy' may be connected with Fernel's expressed opinion, reported by Plancy, that young physicians mis-spend hours in looking at pictures in anatomy books, when what should be done was to go to actual dissections with a concise manual in the hand. Fernel made his 'Anatomy' a concise manual. It was a preface to his account of the working of the body. Anatomy is to physiology,[3] he says, as geography to history, it describes the theatre of events.

After its anatomy follows the rest of Fernel's treatise, and it is undiluted physiology as then understood. Its books and chapters correspond little with the divisions of the subject to-day. We look in vain for subdivisions such as respiration, digestion, metabolism, etc., let alone circulation. Fernel is writing, of course, eighty years before Harvey's discovery. The divisions we find are: the Elements (*e.s.* the four elements of Empedocles),[4] the Temperaments, the Spirits, the Innate Heat, the Faculties, the Humours, and the Procreation of Man. The anatomical introduction exerts little influence on the arrangement of the treatise. Fernel, earnest man, opens by asking: 'What is the intimate composition of the body?' He had neither chemistry nor microscope. Observer as he is, at this point he says, with a sigh, 'in passing from anatomy to physiology—that is to the actions of the body—we pass from what we can see and feel

1 His directions depart from Galen, *De adm. anat. c.* 2.
2 The Oporinus *De Fabrica* bears on its title-page the same subject as the wood-cut on the title-page of Linacre's *Galeni Medendi Methodus*, issued thirteen years before by de Colines. Van Kalcar's version for the Vesalius has changed the scene into a vulgar Babel of strident curiosity. Fielding Garrison finds it 'reek of the Barnum's show-bill' (*Principles of Anatomical Illustration*).
3 *De Nat. Parte Med.*, praefatio; also peroratio.
4 Fernel attributes them to Hippocrates. *Dialog.* ii, preface.

to what is known only by meditation'.[1] 'The ultimate elements are not to be reached by observation and the senses',[2] but only by cogitation. All the same, although his 'elements' are not accessible to observation, he proceeds to construct the body from them. He seems to forget they are conjecture. His elements are of course those of the ancients, earth, air, fire, water, not indeed as we meet them in the concrete, but as they existed in abstract, in the thought of antiquity, and indeed in the abstract thought of Fernel's own time. They are vehicles for four cardinal 'qualities', dry, wet, warm, cold, on which depended the temperament of man, and of things animate and inanimate. These cardinal qualities are, however, not necessarily to be sensed. They are often potential, not actual. Thus, temperament or 'constitution' consisted of their admixed potentialities. The most sensitive of our thermometers, hygrometers, etc. of to-day would have been powerless to detect either the 'warm' or the 'wet', or their contraries, in so far as they were in potentiality. Moreover, each cardinal element carried, besides its main quality, an accessory quality compatible with its main one, also, it might be, in potentiality.

These four elements and the four qualities had been, for perhaps twenty centuries, a pillar of theoretical medicine. Despite such overwhelming tradition, Fernel has a word to say on his own part in introducing them:[3]

The science of things was at first rough, and turned only on what the eye or ear or other senses could seize. Effects were accepted without thought about them. In time observation penetrated deeper, knowledge got further from the merely sensual, and the abstract was reached. Then first was philosophy born in word and deed—philosophy, which seeks to trace in the manifold the effects of causes, and to bring all together. Much, however, is still obscure. We may smile at the old atoms, and wonder how anyone could be persuaded of them. A number of solid indivisible corpuscles which, by collecting chancewise, have brought to pass the immensity, the variety, the completeness of the manifold of all the adornment of this world. Truly, Democritus, could he be with us again, would still, and even more cynically than ever, smile,[4] as was his wont, at our supposed elements.[5]

1 *Physiol.* ii, praefatio.   2 *Physiol.* ii, 3.   3 *Dialog.* ii, prefatio.
4 *La cause morale du Ris de l'excellent et très-renommè Democrite, expliqué et temoigné par le divin Hippocras, en ses Epitres*, traduit de Grec en Fransais par M. I. Guichard, docteur-regent de l'Univ. Mompelier. Nicol. Chesneau, Paris: au Chesne Verd. rue St Jacques, 1579. Cf. also L. Joubert's *Traité du Ris*.
5 'Multo acrius haec quae putamus elementa, suo more rideret.'

Hippocrates, however, was credited with taking the 'Democritus smile' as one that was wise and kindly. Fernel continues: 'These elements seem established with reasonable probability. Where I want to be clear is that those who accept the four elements, as cause of all which is, are sometimes greatly led away by their own arguments. The causes of many happenings lie elsewhere.'[1] It is true the alchemists took what they called sulphur—the combustible factor, that which disappeared from the crucible—for an element, and again, Cardan[2] argued for three elements only, rejecting 'fire'. But what I think Fernel is referring to, in thus qualifying the theory of the elements, is the 'total substance', of which he treats later in the 'Dialogue' itself.[3]

Fernel then proceeds to 'temperament', that is, the balance of the four cardinal qualities, cold, warm, dry, wet; it constitutes health. A perfect balance, an ideal health, was impossible of attainment. In each individual the temperament inherently leaned a little toward one or other of the cardinal qualities. This inclination was decisive for health, and for disease. The immediate cause of disease was disturbance of the approximately balanced temperament. To judge the 'temperament' of the patient was the physician's first step. The same disease acted differently according to the temperament.[4]

The opening chapter of book iii is entitled 'What the temperament is, and how Avicenna has described it wrongly.' Fernel was impatient of the Arabs; nor was he alone in that. Medicine had 'presented itself to Medieval Christendom in an Arabian dress',[5] but that tendency was wearing itself thin. The 'Arabist' manuals were, it is true, still 'favourites': the Articella, the Practica, the Lilium Medicinae, Rosa Anglica, and so on. They were compact of Avicenna, Mesue, Rhases, etc.; and the practitioner still leaned on them. But already before Fernel's day the tide of Arabic influence was in its ebb. Janus Cornarius, Fernel's contemporary, urged that all the Schools 'should, as the Florentine Academy had done, repudiate the errors of the barbarians'. The library of the physician had been undergoing a significant change. Pierre Cardonnel, Canon of Notre-Dame in Paris, a doctor-

1 Dialog. ii, preface.
2 Vita sua propria, p. 216. Cf. Riolan the elder's De primis principiis rerum nat., bk. i, c. 5, p. 429 (1588).
3 Dialog. ii, c. 10; and cf. supra, p. 37 and p. 52.
4 Cf. Dr Kellett, 'Two Medicines', Medical World, Feb. 9, 1945.
5 J. F. Payne, Galen's De temperamentis, with introduction, Cambridge, 1881.

regent of the Faculty of Medicine for thirty-two years, had a library which on its owner's death, in 1438, came to sale, and its valuation-inventory is extant.[1] Of its twenty-five works on medicine, all but two, a Galen and—if we admit surgery—a Lanfranc, were Arab. As against this, we have the inventory, discovered recently[2] and dating about the year 1500, of the physician Antonio Benivieni—one of the 'signore' of Florence. Among its forty-nine medical volumes there is a leaven of several non-Arab editions of Aristotle and Galen, and further a Celsus and a Pliny. One section of it, however, was completely 'Arab' still, the section labelled by its owner 'astrology'. The anti-Arab attitude of Fernel tells us, just once more, that he belonged in medicine, as in so much else, to the humanist revival, already in his student-time beginning to affect the University of Paris.

But it would be a mistake to suppose that that movement brought a rebirth of medicine, or of the sciences of Nature cognate to medicine. Indeed, some argue to-day that the humanist movement of the fifteenth and sixteenth centuries went with a slackening of advance in medicine and science. Certainly the 'revival of letters' practically ran its course, without either the new Science or the new Medicine appearing. The medical humanists themselves, although adding to the cultural prestige of medicine, did little toward refounding either its art or science. Symphorien Champier, Leonicenus,[3] Linacre,[4] Sylvius, Barbarus, Brasavola, we turn in vain to these for any notable contribution—let alone discovery—advancing medicine. They had not the necessary outlook; their toil spent in commenting on the ancient texts is in itself evidence that they did not possess the point of view. The progress of science—if we seek to allot a date to its actual steps—is nearest related to the *De Revolutionibus*, 1543, of the Polish astronomer, trained in Italy, Copernicus. Even that work passed long with scant notice from either the humanist or the medical world of its time. Astrology went on its way unconcerned by it. Fernel's 'Dialogue', published five years after it, seems unaware of it.

Fernel, at the outset of his book iii, argues the nature of the com-

1 Chereau, A., *Bulletin de Bibliophile*, Paris, 1864.
2 By Professor Bindo de Vecchi, *Bibliofilia*, 34, Florence, 1932; also Ralph M. Major, *Bull. Hist. Med.* III (1935), p. 739.
3 *V. infra*, Note XV, *Appendix*, p. 183.
4 *V. infra*, Note XVI, *Appendix*, p. 184.

bination of the elements in the temperament. Fernel says the elements in the temperament resemble notes in a musical chord.[1] Each note persists in its individuality though merged in the chord. Fernel finds 'absurd' the teaching of Avicenna that, merged in the temperament, the cardinal qualities individually disappear. How, he asks, can that be when, in old age, the cold and dry of the temperament reappear and dominate? They were not destroyed. They were latent, although obscured. Hence we carry in our temperament not only the basis of our health but the seeds of our dissolution. Fernel's scheme was of the type of a mingling of yellow and blue pigments to look green. Avicenna's resembled a firing of hydrogen and oxygen, when the gases disappear and water replaces them. Fernel's doctrine seems the better suited for teaching the 'humoral' medicine of his time.

Medical tradition, it is said, had, even before the Hippocratic writings, identified with the four cardinal elements and their qualities, four so-called cardinal 'humours' in the body. They were the 'blood', equivalent to air, hot and moist; the 'yellow bile' or choler to fire, hot and dry; the 'phlegm' (pituita), which included the supposed secretion of the brain through the nose, to water, moist and cold; the 'black bile' (melancholy) to earth, dry and cold. Excess of one of these in the temperament caused an idiosyncrasy of the temperament, and such idiosyncrasies were classified according to the particular ingredient dominant. It was a habit already ingrained in medicine to use the humours for designating the temperaments. A patient was classed as melancholic, or sanguine, or phlegmatic, or choleric, or as inclining to pairs of these. The terms themselves had passed beyond medicine into everyday speech. They still survive there. But Fernel objected to them as lax expression. He took his theoretical medicine too strictly to condone them. He says [2] 'we may speak of a temperament as hot, or moist, or hot-moist, and so on, but it is wrong to call it sanguine, though this is commonly done'. It is wrong because the four humours, e.g. the blood and the others, are not strictly parts of the living body. They are merely contained *in* the body. They themselves are not alive. Moreover, he adds, experience every day disproves that the humours compose the temperament. Touch is, after all, the practical criterion for temperament; often the fair and plump, judged by the touch, are cool, and this though they have abundance of good blood. Their temperament is cool and dry, despite their blood which is warm and moist. Such people are of sanguine humour, but not of sanguine temperament. To call them of sanguine temperament is worse than meaningless; it is misleading.

Fernel turns to the three coctions, part of the very marrow of contemporary medical teaching. By the first coction was meant the conversion of food into chyle. The second or 'great' coction was that which manufactured the blood, the chief of the four humours. The third coction, broadly taken, was the becoming flesh of the material absorbed from the veins, called omoiesis. Fernel does not, however, proceed to the three coctions, until after he has (in book v) spoken of the 'faculties of the soul'.[1] That may seem strange, but it was logical. The faculties of the psyche were 'causes'—in this case, of the coctions. That primary faculty, the 'nutritive', worked the first coction. It did so by means of the 'natural spirits' as agent. These spirits acted on the temperaments of the foods and of the organs concerned with the foods. Medical doctrine likened the processes of the first and second coctions to cooking, whence the name 'coction'. The natural heat assisted this cooking, but, Fernel said, the innate heat, not the elemental heat. This heat is concentrated so as to resemble a fire put under a cauldron.[2] Fernel says that a finger inserted into the left ventricle of an animal's heart finds it the warmest point in the whole body[3]—perhaps he knew the observation at first hand.

Food should be of good 'temperament'. The change alters it beyond mere change of qualities; the change is of its very substance.[4] Fernel is not satisfied that the coctions *are* simply cooking. The first coction may be so. But there are difficulties; the first coction of the ostrich dissolves iron, which even the hottest lion cannot dissolve. The lion was famed for its hot temperament. Again, the quail eats hellebore, without hurt, though hellebore, even after cooking, poisons a strong man. Nicolas Oresme,[5] the shrewd-minded Bishop of Lisieux, had asked in the fourteenth century how it was that fish, which have no warmth, can perform the coction of food. Fernel similarly wonders how shellfish do so, seeing they have neither warmth nor blood. It was perhaps to overcome these difficulties he declared the heat employed was the 'innate heat'—not the 'elemental'.

1 The 'faculties' were by some traced to 'virtues' of the celestial motions; cf. Paparella, *De Calido*, ii, c. 13 and c. 17, Perugia, 4°, 1573.
2 *Physiol.* vi, c. 1.   3 *Physiol.* iii, c. 6.
4 *De purgatione*, iii, p. 12.
5 L. Thorndike, *History of Magic and Experimental Science*, III, p. 464.

At the same time he demurs from the opinion held by some of the ancients [1]—not by Aristotle—that the first coction is a putrefaction. He says a sort of brew is produced, namely the chyme; this, though not pleasant to the taste, is yet wholesome, for the stomach accepts it. He adds,[2] 'some teach that this chyme is what the stomach lives on, but the stomach like the rest of the body takes its nutriment from the blood in its own veins. And, lest my contradiction seem merely empty and vexatious, I ask how in the womb does the stomach of the child which has veins but no chyme get its nourishment except through its veins?' 'In the intestine the veins suck up chyme as the roots of a tree suck juice from the earth.'[3]

Fernel's remarks on the passage of food from the mouth to the stomach strongly suggest he had actually seen the transit exposed to view, possibly by some injury. He says the food does not simply run down into the stomach; it is grasped by the back of the mouth and gullet 'as by a hand'.[4] The gullet, above the morsel, contracts on it and drives it down, while below the morsel the gullet dilates and sucks it. This is exactly true and waited until the nineteenth century for re-discovery by Angelo Mosso, of Turin. And a similar push-pull process obtains in the intestine, as discovered by the Viennese Nothnagel. Helpful to the surgeon for detecting, when the intestine is laid bare in an abdominal operation, which is the upper and which the lower end of a coil, it became known in the nineteenth century as 'Nothnagel's sign'. Fernel also states, as if he had actually seen it, that the stomach while churning its contents keeps its lower opening tight for a time. John de Mirfeld, the priest attached to St Bartholomew's Hospital, London, remarks[5] that criminals hanging by their heels still take food and drink.

What the stomach does, as he describes it, is explained by Fernel[6] by calling in three sub-faculties, 'attractive', 'concoctive' and 'expulsive' respectively; divisions of the great 'nutritive faculty'. A faculty was an 'efficient cause', and even much later than Fernel.[7] Two further 'causes' operating digestion are the 'alterative' faculty

1 *Physiol.* (1542), p. 109 recto.   2 *Physiol.* vi, c. i.
3 *Ibid.* c. 2.   4 *Physiol.* (1542) p. 127b.
5 MS. in British Museum, *Breviarium Bartholomei*, see *Johannes de Mirfeld of St Bartholomew's, Smithfield:, his Life and Works*, by Sir P. Horton-Smith Hartley and H. R. Aldridge, 1936, Camb. Univ. Press.
6 *Physiol.* vi, c. 1.
7 Le Verduc, *Le Maistre de Chirurgie*, 1709.

and the 'commutative'. Hunger, the sensation, resides in the wall of the stomach. When food arrives, the stomach experiences pleasure (*voluptas*). In due course it transmits the food onward to other organs, in order that they as well may profit. But that does not, Fernel says, justify our thinking the stomach endowed with reason and intelligence, although a certain care and foresight are shown. All we can allow is that, having got its fill, it disburdens itself of the rest, and does so with a will.[1] Evidently for Fernel a mind of a sort is immanent in these organs.

The product of the first coction, the chyle, is taken to the liver by the veins of the intestine. The veins have tiny side openings, 'oscula', too small to be visible. Through these the body everywhere sucks nutriment from the veins. The cause which operates this is the faculty 'attractrix'. It has selective power; thus, it takes in white wine more quickly than red.[2] Fernel was perplexed as to the route by which the chyle travels to the liver. The chyle is white, the veins contain red blood. 'A thorny question, not open to the court of the senses.' He wonders whether some veins carry chyle, others blood. He is thus asking for the 'lacteals', eighty years before Aselli found them. He concludes that the chyle must be mixed with the blood in the veins.

As to the great second coction, its seat lies in the liver. It manufactures the blood (*procreatio sanguinis*). This, Fernel argues, is *not* like a cooking process, though it may well require the vital heat. But it is not the heat which does it. It is some power intrinsic in the liver.[3] He declares the process resembles *fermentation*. Descartes seems here to have read Fernel.[4] The chyle, after being poured into the liver, is there fermented. Something like the deposit in a must-vat forms, and something light, like the floating 'flower' of the must-vat. The former is the black bile, the melancholy, the humour which goes to the spleen to be stored. The latter is the yellow bile, the choler, which is stored in the bile-cyst under the liver. Fernel denies that any kitchen-like chambers exist in the liver. The actual substance of the liver is the fashioner of the blood (*opifex sanguinis*). Fernel therefore, in the mid-sixteenth century, when the theme of fermentation turned chiefly round the alchemical production of gold, was stressing it as

1 *Physiol.* v, c. 9, p. 129. It is interesting to compare Fernel in all this with the great modern experimenter, Ivan Pavlov, *Researches on Digestion*, transl. by W. H. Thompson, London.

2 *Physiol.* vi, c. 2, p. 131; Galen, *De Nat. Facult.* iii, at end.

3 *Ibid.* III, c. 3, pp. 133 b, 134 a.   4 *De Homine*, III, p. 4, 1662.

the process by which the liver produces the blood and the bile. The liver is known to-day to be a hive of ferments.

From the liver the new-made blood is carried to all parts by the great *vena cava* and its branches. The liver is the beginning of the whole venous system.[1] Fernel asks what drives the blood from the liver along the whole venous tree, out to the uttermost ends of the body? He says it cannot be the heart because when blood flows from a vein it shows no pulse. The blood must be attracted outward along the veins by all the parts which need it (*facultas attractrix*). Each part sucks in what it wants. This suction causes the blood next upstream to move, giving additively the whole flow from the liver outward. Harvey was, of course, to show that the direction of movement is exactly opposite to that fancied by Fernel and his time. To enter into Fernel's position we have to rid our mind of the notion, which now seems almost self-evident, that blood flows *through* the liver.[2] The blood did not, for those of Fernel's time, flow *through* any organ. That it could do so would never have entered Fernel's or any other head of that period.[3]

The third coction converted material, drawn from the veins by the flesh, into the substance of that flesh, of whatsoever kind. Fernel was puzzled as to how the particular matter destined for each particular part got thither. No Harveian circulation yet helped to elucidate that. Fernel invoked a special cause, a 'faculty'. Resort of that kind was common enough; the *facultas attractrix* was at hand. For the converse difficulty—removal of the unwanted—he called in a *facultas expultrix*. These examples of the *deus ex machina* were not of Fernel's invention. They were stock-in-trade of the time. Philiatros,[4] in the 'Dialogue', speaks of faculties as explanations to which the physician makes appeal. He adds that Averrhoes considers the faculties to be separate souls.[5] Fernel employed them as causes. 'The gall-bladder attracts the yellow bile from the liver through a special duct. Its bile is pure and unmixed with any other humour, partly because the tenuity of the channel keeps back coarser material, but mainly because the attraction rests on kinship and preternatural accord (*familiaritate*

1 *Physiol.* i, c. 11, p. 32, v, c. 14, p. 101: 'Jecur venarum esse originē hic prohypothesi constituam, cujus tamen veritatem' etc.
2 *Physiol.* i, c. 11: 'Vena cava non est continuata venis mesenterii.'
3 Servetus, however, had the idea of blood traversing the lung, in his *Restitutio Christianismi*, of eleven years later than Fernel's 'Physiology'.
4 *Dialog.* ii, c. 5, p. 473.   5 Cf. S. Paparella, *op. cit.* i, c. xiii.

et occulta convenientia) with the humour. The humour, though sharp and acrid, is not hostile to its own proper receptacle, rather it is blithe and friendly by mutual affinity, so that the receptacle experiences a satisfaction and a certain pleasure.[1] This is all of a piece with an organic mind diffused in the organs, as we saw in the case of the hunger in the wall of the stomach. The mechanical problem of the storage of bile is thus satisfied by a supposed psychical sympathy between the chamber of storage and the fluid stored. We are back in that past age whence Schopenhauer recruited later his mythical 'will-to-live'.

Most of Fernel's physiology is orthodox medical tradition current in his time, but it presents points of originality. He demurs from Aristotle's notion that in the body the blood remains unclotted because it is there kept warm. Fernel argues that the veins exercise restraint over clotting. This was a point stressed by Lister, the surgeon, only last century, from observations of his own. As to the relative quantities of the four humours in the blood, Fernel, lover of numeration, may have itched to give them. Their proportions are sometimes written in on the margin of his page by some zealous reader. Their variability in fact made such numbers an insincerity which perhaps Fernel would not countenance.

In Fernel's time the heart had not yet acquired the importance in medicine which has attached to it since Harvey's discovery. In regard to it Fernel largely follows the orthodox description then current, but he gives it with a clearness all his own. We cite it here, condensed. The heart has two chambers, one right, one left (the auricles were not reckoned as parts of the heart proper). The right and left in all phases of their action synchronize. The phase of dilatation is active, and draws blood from the great stem vein, *vena cava*, into the right chamber, and 'prepared air' from the lung into the left chamber through the venous artery (pulmonary vein). This active dilatation, 'called in greek diastole', opens the valve at entrance to each chamber, and shuts the valves at exit of each chamber, namely at the root of the great artery and at the root of the arterial vein entering the lung. The direction of these heart-valves is described in confirmation of this. In succession to this suction-pump phase (diastole) follows the force-pump phase (systole), in which the chambers actively contract in size. This phase in the right chamber shuts the valve guarding the great vein that the suction-phase had opened, and opens the valves

---

1 *Physiol.* vi, c. 3, p. 134 a (c. 4 of the 1554 and later editions).

at the arterial vein to the lung; into this latter it drives blood for the nourishment of the lung—this does not imply a conception that any blood passes *through* the lung. Similarly, in the heart's left chamber; the valve from the lung which the suction-phase had opened is shut at systole, the valves guarding the great artery are opened, and blood is driven into that artery and its branches—blood charged with compressed vital spirit. The charging of the blood with spirit has been done in the left-side heart-chamber, the spirit there being elaborated from the prepared air sucked from the lung by the active expansion (diastole) of the chamber. The walls of the great artery and its branches are specially thick to prevent leakage of the spirit through them.

To this Fernel adds an observation of importance which seems original with him. It is [1] that at the moment when the ventricles shrink in size (systole) the arteries *increase* in size. The teaching of the day was the contrary of this; it taught, namely, that 'the moment of occurrence of increase in volume of the arteries coincided with that of the increase in volume (diastole) of the ventricle. Descartes' *De Homine*, one hundred years later than Fernel, still states so. Fernel, after making his statement, remarks that this expansion of the arteries which accompanies the shrinkage of the ventricle is caused by the ventricle's systole forcing into them the mixture of blood and compressed spirit which the ventricle contains. Fernel seems the first to make this observation and this comment, tracing expansion of the arteries to injection by the ventricle. They are sometimes attributed to Caesalpino's *Quaestiones peripateticae*, v, 4, 1571, or to Realdo Columbo, in the *De Re Anatomica*, 1559.[2] But Fernel's observation was published in 1542, and had appeared in five editions (Paris, Lyons, Venice) before Columbo's book appeared, and in three more (Frankfort) before Caesalpino's.

The travel of the pulse outward along the arteries was too quick for Fernel's inspection to detect—as also later for Descartes. He remarks: 'It is not however entirely by the supply of inflowing blood and spirits that the arteries are expanded; they would not then pulsate *throughout their length at the same moment*. It would be impossible for the spirits and blood in a moment to travel along to the furthest ends of the arteries.'[3] He gives the arteries an active expansive diastole

1 *Physiol.* vi, c. 18.
2 R. A. Young, *Harveian Oration*, London, 1939, p. 13.
3 *Physiol.* vi, c. 18.

of their own like that of the heart, and of simultaneous occurrence throughout their length, alternating with that of the heart. This active diastole of the arteries, timed alternately with that of the heart, was followed by an active arterial systole. We may think it would have been simpler to suppose it a phase of elastic recoil on the part of the stretched artery, when, the distending force over, the vessel partly empties itself again. But for Fernel and his time there was no *distal escape* of blood from the artery into the veins (*via* the capillaries). There was no distal exit through which the artery could empty itself. Knowledge of that came only with Harvey. What Fernel supposed was that between the successive distensions of the artery by the heart's systole an active systole of the artery compressed the spirits and drove off from them 'sooty' impurities.[1] The blood and spiritus did not so much move onward as suffer compression. This helped to squeeze a supply of them through 'oscula' in the vessel-wall, thus helping to feed the organs; which, however, were chiefly nourished from the veins. The greater thickness of the arterial wall than the venous, like the greater thickness of the left ventricle than the right, was a device for preventing too free escape of the tenuous 'spirits' mixed with the arterial blood.

The scale of the blood flow was for a time, even by those who accepted the circulation, much underrated. Harvey's estimate was that the heart at each stroke drives into the great artery (aorta) 2 ounces of blood. Riolan fils opposed Harvey because he could not suppose so large a blood-flow through the lungs. The *Marrow of Surgery*, an excellent manual,[2] adopting the new discovery as early as 1647, says, of the blood, its 'motion is universal, continual, vehement, swift alike in veins and arteries, so that the whole blood being 24 pound, passeth through a circulation, some say in three hours, others in twenty-four'. The time varies much with different degrees of bodily activity. The *Marrow of Surgery*'s circumspect estimate of several hours has in fact in some conditions to be reduced to less than a minute. Descartes, in the *De Homine* (1662), accepting the circulation, speaks of the blood returning to the heart 'drop by drop'.[3] But in violent exercise a volume of blood five times the whole of that within the body may race through the heart each minute. One effect of Harvey's discovery was that the arteries began to assume an importance in medicine equal

---

1 *Pathol.* iii, c. I.   2 By James Cook of Warwick, surgeon.
3 *De Homine*, III, p. 5.

76

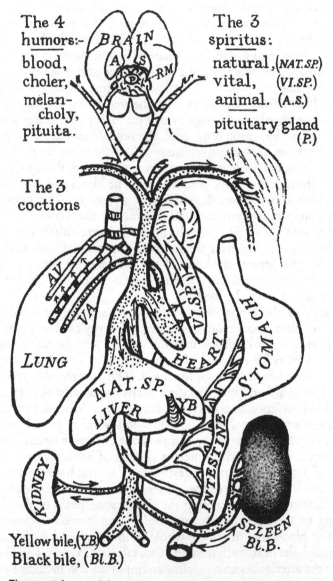

The 4
humors:-
blood,
choler,
melan-
choly,
pituita.

The 3
spiritus:
natural, (NAT.SP.)
vital, (VI.SP.)
animal. (A.S.)

pituitary gland
(P.)

The 3
coctions

BRAIN

A *S*

RM

AV

VA

VI.SP.

LUNG

HEART

STOMACH

NAT. SP.

LIVER

YB

INTESTINE

KIDNEY

SPLEEN
Bl.B.

Yellow bile, (Y.B)
Black bile, (Bl.B.)

Fig. 13. Scheme of the organs of the Galenical 'vital faculty'.

to that of the veins. The heart itself, which had been chiefly the prime seat of all fever, became the most urgently necessary organ of all bodily life.

As to the 'cause' of the heart's movements, and of the active pulse of the arteries, Fernel rates them as sub-faculties of the *vital* faculty. They ally themselves to the rhythmic motions of the lungs—and brain. Hence it is that the heart, the arteries and the lungs stand together as the '*vital* parts'.[1] The '*vital* faculty' is distinguished from the '*natural* faculty' by reason of the operations of the '*natural* faculty' being nutritional and not exhibiting movement. Those of the animal faculty are characterized by movement which can be made or

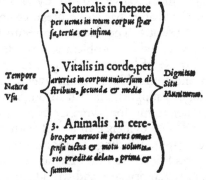

Fig. 14. Précis of faculties: 'facultates corpus nostrum dispensantes, in quibus est nostra vita, sunt tres'. J. Sylvius, in Linacre's Galen, Paris, 1537, 2°.

restrained by the will, and are subject to fatigue. But the *vital* movements are not made by the will and are not subject to fatigue.[2] For that reason Fernel[3] does not count the heart a *muscle*.

Fernel treats mind as coming within physiology.[4] It forms the theme of a full third of his 'Physiology'. He includes the mind and its workings within physiology not because he regards the mental as an affair of matter. That was not his conception at all. *Res incorporeae sunt objecta intelligentiae.* He considered the action of the mind a part of physiology because for him all the workings which went on in the body were, at source, non-material and incorporeal. The coctions, the motions of the heart, the movements of the limbs, were, even as

1 *Physiol.* i, c. 8, p. 24.   2 *Physiol.* iv, c. 13, p. 116.
3 *Physiol.* i, c. 8.   4 *Physiol.* v, c. 1.

much as were thoughts in the brain, traceable to an immaterial soul operating the body. The mental was just one among the activities of that soul. The living body did not even live *of its own self*; it was made to live by the immaterial life-soul within it. The life-soul was one and indivisible, though with faculties for doing this and that. In this Fernel continues much which had gone before. In the 'Physiology'[1] he says: 'In all animate beings, and most in man, the body has been created for the sake of the soul (*gratia animae*). It is for that soul not only a habitation (*diversorium*) but an adjusted instrument for use by its (the soul's) inherent powers.' Figard[2] finds a difference between Aquinas and Fernel in the former describing the matter of the body as simple brute matter made to live and 'do' by the soul within, while Fernel teaches that the matter has to be prepared in order that the soul may vivify and use it.[3] The distinction seems to indicate that Fernel feels himself faced with a problem and is wrestling with it.

With Fernel and those of his time, along with assumption of the intervention of a life-soul ubiquitous in every act of the body, there went an analogous supposition, that throughout the vast manifold of being every active motion, whether of plant or animal, even of the humblest kind, was evidence of a soul within which *felt* and *willed*. Thus Fernel imputed feeling, memory, desire, fancy, to the very lowliest creatures known to him. He says the oyster and other shellfish shrink away when pricked, and would run off if they could. Every creature finds in the world some things pleasant and others unpleasant.[4] Every creature has a certain measure of imagination and reflection (*fingendi cogitandique facultas*). Each seeks the pleasant and avoids the unpleasant. The pleasant excites an agitation in the mind compelling 'appetition' toward it. In man only is this controllable by a 'will which is free'.

'Feeling' and 'will' were thus injected into life's simplest types. Schopenhauer, even as late as last century, harked back to that demonological view, and even with exaggeration. In the 'Dialogue' Fernel accounts for the behaviour of iron and the magnet by an animate 'sympathy' between the two, akin to a desire of the soul. A century later than Fernel the occultist chemist, Stahl, attributed the writhing of a scrap of hide seared by a hot iron to the act of the

---

1 Bk. i, c. 2 of 1554. The chapter was partly rewritten from the original edition (1542); this sentence had a prototype there, but is not textually the same.

2 *Jean Fernel*, p. 161.   3 *Dialog.* i, c. 5, toward end.

4 *Physiol.* v, cc. 6, 9.

'rational soul' within the hide. Not until 1649 were the words of detachment and reason spoken. Then René Descartes issued some famous 'articles' in the *Passions de l'Âme*. They denied that the body's doings were the work of a 'spirit' within it, and asserted most of its doings to be doings done by itself.

Fernel's 'Physiology', proceeding with its account of the mind, treats mind and brain together. Any question as to 'how' mind and brain work together seems not to present itself. The brain 'refines' the animal spirits gradually; purged at last of all corporeal dross, they become concepts, finally even universal concepts, and ideas of the moral 'values'. These successive purifications require the 'internal motions'[1] of the brain. The raw 'species' and 'simulacra' and 'spectra' of sense are at outset far from free of gross matter. On their arrival at the 'common sensorium' further purification begins. What passes thence to the passive intellect is cleansed of dross further

bus, quā ratione vna fit &   mentis 105.20. locus de fe
simplex   213.6   mine   138.33
Animã nō eſſe ſimplicē, qui- Ariſtotelis locus de vi attra-
bus argumētis ſuadet 213.30   ctrice ſtirpium   174.36
Animam noſtrã eſſe immor-   Ars   195.9,& 274.28
talem   214.30   Arteria maior ἀορτὴ dicta 42.
Animæ actiones læduntur læ   Arteriarũ vſus 68.26   (37

Fig. 15. Item from Index of the *De Naturali Parte Medicinae* 1542.

still. After a series of refinings, that which reaches the active intellect is practically free from earthliness. Reason itself is ultimately relieved from every trace of the corporeal and earthly, and is free to think and will, and is fit for immortality.

Fernel is careful to maintain that the soul, despite its different faculties, is one. The triple soul of Plato he rejects. It would endanger his faith's doctrine of immortality. The soul is one. The soul is utterly simple. It cannot be split. It cannot be subdivided. It is an individuum, a spiritual unity. It cannot be dismembered. If it cannot come to pieces, disintegration cannot overwhelm it; it cannot perish. It is immortal.[2] In the table of contents of his 'Physiology' there occurs, attaching to the item 'soul', 'that our soul is immortal'.[3] 'Though the manifestations of the soul are multiple the soul itself is one. The different, and even opposed, functions of the several parts of the body do not mean a multiple soul.' Here Fernel's religious

---

1 *Physiol.* vi, c. 10 and 14.   2 *Physiol.* v, c. 18.

3 'Anima: nostram animam immortalem esse': still so in the revised ultimate (Geneva, 1680) edition.

faith is struggling against Alexander Aphrodisias, who, he says, has misinterpreted Aristotle. 'The different functions of different parts of the body come from the differently prepared nature of those material parts (organs) in which the one and single soul is diffused. It is as when one and the same craftsman uses different tools.' There is a passage where Fernel has resort to the old simile which likened the rational soul in the body to a pilot in his boat. That was one of the heresies later alleged against Giordano Bruno.[1] He mentions it not wholly to endorse it. To make clearer to us his conception of death, he himself offers a simile. It was something he wished to insist on, for he gives it twice.[2] He writes: 'Look you, suppose a craftsman with whom all goes well. He is inside a room. To do the work which seems to him good he needs his tools. And he needs light that he may see. So it is with the soul. While within the trammels of the body, the soul, in order that it may understand and reason, needs a fit place and usable things. If these fail, it works no more and quits.' The life-soul, so to say, goes on strike. Fernel was probably the greatest physician of his century. This simile of his seems to carry us with him to the bedside of the dying. There, doubtless many times, he stood with that homely poignant simile in his mind. For him the problem with which he would then be faced was to refit, to reillumine, the darkening chamber, which otherwise its occupant, the distressed soul, would quit.

We said that Fernel seems not to apprehend any difficulty about the spiritual and the corporeal (the material) interacting. Rather perhaps any difficulty he has does not present itself to him in that way. He says: 'The parts and organs of the body are only instruments of the soul and of its faculties, and without those parts and organs the soul and its faculties could not do their work. Although instruments are all that those parts and organs are, we yet cannot avoid treating them as though they were immediate causes, and that is so because the substance of the soul and of its faculties is deeply hidden from us.'[3] Fernel had of course Galen's 'spirits' to serve as mediators between the corporeal and incorporeal, much as astrology had the 'astral fluid' to serve as medium for occult influences of a star in stellar action on sublunary things. Fernel is at times careful to classify these 'spirits' which mediate between soul and flesh.

1 V. Spampanato, *Documenti d. Vita di Giordano Bruno*, Florence, 1933, p. 182.
2 *Dialog.* ii, c. 4; *Physiol.* v, c. 18.
3 *Pathol.* i, c. 3.

The original provenance of Galen's animal spirits is, by some, traced to Plato's *Timaeus*: 'When the eyelids close, they confine the fire within them, and it diffuses and quiets the movements within.'[1] This 'fire', it is thought, may have suggested the 'animal spirits'. The association seems a little far to seek. Galen's three sorts of spirits—natural (πνεῦμα φυσικόν), vital (ζωτικόν) and animal (ψυχικόν); Fernel says the 'vital' are aerial, the 'animal' etherial—had come to be a birthright of the medieval and of the Renaissance physician. Fernel comments on the term 'spirit' as 'meaning in all languages "air" or "breath"'; although invisible, producing effects. In that respect it is akin both to the corporeal and the incorporeal. It is therefore of an intermediate category. Everything which is incorporeal and escapes our sense and yet exerts influence upon us and on corporeal objects does so by means of spirit.'[2] The 'natural' spirits were intermediaries for the nutritive operations of the life-soul; a sort of half-way house between substance of soul and material of body. It was as though matter, poured out thin, lost some of its materiality. To-day physical science, our expert on the subject of matter, disallows any half-way house between the material and the non-material. For Fernel the 'image' in the eyeball entering the brain as 'animal spirits' became, in the latter, a thought, and the transmutation asked no comment.

In treating of our muscular movements, and their relation to our thinking, Fernel makes in passing a notable remark, not met with in the customary handling of the subject. It is that some of our acts occur quite apart from 'appetition' and 'will'. Some movements of the eyes and eyelids, and of the head, and also of the hands during sleep, and again our movements of breathing, do not proceed, he says, from intent or any other impulse of the mind; they lie outside the mind. Thus he distinguishes a category of active muscular movement independent of will, or other intention—pure 'motricity' acting of itself. Fernel does not elaborate this further. But in the following century, whether unaware of Fernel's remark or not, Descartes returned to similar observations, and dealt with them in a manner which caught the abiding attention of the world.

Fernel comes presently to Aristotle's 'common sensorium'. There the mind receives, compares, distinguishes and sorts out the arriving

1 Stephan, 45.   2 *Dialog.* ii, c. 7.

sensual images and simulacra. Without this sifting, man's thought could do little with them. Fernel's brevity and vigour picture the images and simulacra crowding in upon a recipient and percipient soul. It might seem natural, in describing such a scene, to stage the recipient soul as central figure and to identify it explicitly with the 'self'. The notion of 'self' attaches to it indisputably as active receptionist of the incomers to its house. Such a view of the scene which he is depicting does not occur to, or, if it does, does not interest, Fernel. In missing it, he misses perhaps a half of all which occupies psychology to-day. Its recognition was reserved for the great innovator of a hundred years later, Descartes, with his assertion that his own experiencing was, to himself, sitting as judge, the best certificate of his own being: 'I think, therefore I am.' In short he took consciousness to be direct evidence of the 'self', without need of transit through sense-organs, and without risk of certain frailties of sense. If it be said the proposition is pleonastic and mere tautology, and that all which is rightly assertable is 'there is thinking' and that this does not suffice the argument, his answer might be that the evidence he puts in lies in the very fact that the proposition *is* tautological and cannot but be tautological.[1] Descartes adduces 'thinking' as subjectively experienced—not thinking as objectively observed, this latter being at best sensual inference. By taking subjective experience he short-circuits sense and inferences from sense, with their uncertainties. Quite aside from ways through sense, the 'self' experiences the 'self' directly. Descartes rests his argument on the experiencer as inalienably present in his own experience. He takes this 'subjective self', or first-hand self, as proof to itself of its own existence, and it was to himself that the question about existence had been addressed. He takes it that his 'proof' is applicable to other men besides himself. It may not be applicable to all modes of existence, but to our mode of existence it is. That however apart, Descartes was here, in stressing the 'I', ushering in an element of the modern period.

Fernel proceeds with his account of the mind as begetter of acts. He raises muscular movement to the status of a separate faculty of the life-soul—a faculty of 'motricity'. Aristotle had not so regarded it; for him animal acts always started out from some activity of the mind, e.g. were secondary to sense, and motricity *per se* was not a primary attribute of life. We have to remember that by 'muscles'

1 Cf. also K. W. Monsarrat, p. 39: 'Myself, my thinking and my thoughts', 1942.

Fernel understood only what are spoken of as the voluntary muscles. By 'movements' Fernel means those by the 'voluntary' muscles, for instance, those trains of acts which throughout our waking day constitute to an observer our behaviour. Fernel attributed these movements wholly to a spirit-tenant inside the body.

Descartes broke with this conception—namely, of the body as a puppet worked by a spirit within it. The *Passions de l'Âme*[1] suddenly liquidated this spirit, the *anima* of tradition. The body, it said, is machinery, which does what it does, not in virtue of a spirit-soul in it, but because the outside world releases triggers of the wound-up machinery. Our acts are mechanical reactions started by jostlings against the material world around. Our material microcosm is touched into action by the material macrocosm around it. Descartes, as mathematical physicist, had dealt similarly with the motions of the heavens. He had transferred their operation from a supernatural unmoved prime-mover to matter and natural mechanics. As he dispensed with the immaterial prime-mover in the heavens, so now he dispensed with the immaterial life-soul within the body. 'It is', he said, 'an error to suppose that the soul supplies the body with its heat and its movements.'[2] 'We ought to attribute to our soul (*anima*) no act of ours except our thoughts.'[3] And he went on to say that the death of the body is not owing to the flight of a life-soul from it, but is in fact corporeal breakdown brought about by disintegration of some material organ important to the body.[4]

This pronouncement had a large effect on a large audience. It meant a new freedom in looking at bodily life. It put forward a truth which came to stay. The Renaissance and humanism had as yet brought no such message. It was a message presaging a fresh future for the study of living things, and of medicine. What Descartes styled in brief mechanism would resolve itself, when chemistry and physics grew fuller, into chemistry and physics displacing the occult. But this thesis that the body is the mainspring of its own motions was slow in getting across—even to the physician as physician. In the latter part of the eighteenth century, Haller's full treatise on physiology—seven volumes—makes no mention of 'reflex action', that part of motor behaviour mediated according to Descartes

1 Amsterdam, 1649, London, 1650.   2 *Passions de l'Âme*, art. 5.
3 *Ibid.* art. 17.   4 *Ibid.* art. 6.

by nerves but not actuated by 'reason' or 'will', and called 'reflex'. The notion of reflex action is traceable to Descartes, but the term hardly so. The term is traced more clearly to Thomas Willis. Descartes did not consider all our acts to be 'reflex'. A modicum of our acts he parented upon 'reason' and 'will'. Our 'reflex' behaviour consisted, he taught, of all behaviour which we have in common with animals—animals he thought wholly reflex.

Amateur of the anatomy of man and the domestic animals, Descartes was at pains to provide an anatomical scheme for his mechanism of motor behaviour. This scheme takes us back to Fernel. Descartes was intrigued by valves, perhaps through the part they played in Harvey's discovery of the circulation. The brain when during life exposed to view is seen to rise and fall rhythmically, that is swell and shrink, in the skull. The movement is a passive one, its rhythm is that of the taking of breath; in the seventeenth century it was still supposed to be an activity of the brain itself. Now the brain, despite its look of solidity, is a hollow organ; it has in it four large chambers containing watery fluid. Tradition regarded these as the reservoirs of the Galenical 'spirits', which were generated at the base of the brain. The movement of the brain was taken to be the rhythmic charging of these reservoirs with 'spirits'. The fourth chamber, the hindmost, communicates with the three chambers in front by a narrow tunnel. The entrance to this tunnel is overhung by a small stalked gland. Certain anatomists taught that this gland acted as a valve controlling the passing of spirits backwards and forwards through the tunnel. Fernel himself took that view, describing how the expansion of the brain must raise the gland and free the passage, and the shrinking of the brain must allow the glandular valve to drop into place again and block the tunnel. The valve thus controlled the ebb and flow of spirits to the nerves of all parts. This view was not new. It existed already in the tenth century, in the *Soul and Spirit* of Costa ben Luca, latinized two centuries later by John of Spain, the physician who became Pope. The old tractate attributes the stooping habit of the head when thinking to an effect of that posture being to open the tunnel by lifting the valve. Descartes adopted this gland, and its traditional valvular action, as a key-structure for his scheme. It lay centrally in the brain, and a further supposition, current in Descartes' time, identified the gland with the 'common sensorium' of Aristotle, making it a point of confluence of the animal spirits, coming hither and going thence in all directions. A control valve at such a meeting-place fitted the scheme which Descartes had in mind.

The bodily mechanism of animals and of ourselves, in so far as our ways resemble theirs, Descartes pictured as a complex many-wheeled clock. Different trains of wheels did different things, but all were potentially connected. His supreme central valve controlled their total operation—this little stalked gland, delicately, suspended as he supposed it was, was shiftable in various degrees and directions. Its shifting shunted the running machinery, and the flow of the spirits to and from various parts. The spirits streaming inward from the several sense-organs could deflect the valve. The play of the external world therefore caused movements and changes of movement in the body. When agents of the external world, acting on the nerves, moved the valve, the resulting behaviour was reflex. But the mind also could move the valve and then the behaviour would be 'rational' and the act be one of 'will'. With the latter there went 'conscious ideation'; with the former nothing which Descartes judged truly mental. In placing the valve under the control of events of the mental category (reason, will) Descartes ran against a difficulty. He had laid down that motion in the material universe is fixed in quantity, and he had also laid down that the mind is incorporeal and not material. To assume that the incorporeal mind could move the material valve was to assume an intermeddling between it and the material universe. The universe's motion would then no longer be a fixed quantity— a contradiction to his own postulate.

Time has gradually confirmed Descartes' view that the body's acts are its own. For fuller demonstration more chemistry and physics were required than were available to Descartes. A striking example of physical mechanism operating the body had recently been furnished by Harvey's account of the heart and the circulation of the blood. Descartes saw in the body's ordinary movements, and trains of movements, examples of this same thesis. He held many of them to be wholly independent of thought and mind—to be what is now called 'reflex'. To-day it is established that, in the dog and cat, acts and trains of acts, such as walking, standing, running, galloping, holding a hurt foot from the ground, falling on the feet, shaking and grooming the coat, getting up from lying down, turning the gaze, etc. can all be done under circumstances which preclude the presence of anything we can call 'thoughts'. Descartes' 'robot' behaviour in animals is to this extent demonstrated. So too in considerable measure in ourselves. When, as after spinal injury, some region of the body is deprived of nervous connection with the 'higher' parts of the brain, it becomes a scene of reflex acts resembling those observable in the dog. But in the normal behaviour of the dog, a larger share of behaviour is 'reflex' than in man. And as we descend the animal scale, we meet forms, where the whole of the behaviour would seem to be, even as Descartes supposed, reflex. Man is the most 'mental' of creatures. In him the destruction of those parts of the brain which are associated with recognizable mind leaves little that most of us possibly would dignify by the name of behaviour; no social behaviour would remain to him at all. What does remain to him are these reflexes, of the same type, but not so perfect, as in the dog.

We ask what then of mind in those types of life, countlessly numerous, which are in their organization remote from ours, even to the degree of being wholly devoid of nerve? The animalcule, the vibrio, amoeba, paramaecium. In no single-celled organism is there found what can be thought of as 'nerve'. Such lives cannot therefore have reflex action. Can they, despite that, have recognizable mind? Their ways seem explicable wholly by chemistry and physics. Their chemistry and physics get them their living. There is no need, or room, to complicate interpretation of these lives by supposing a psyche in them. To assume in them the presence of the psychical is an unwarrantable redundancy of 'causes'. Schopenhauer's 'will-to-live' is an instance of that error. It was a return, in the nineteenth century, to the folklore of the Middle Ages. It figured the 'Whole Duty of Man' in the behaviour of an amoeba. In a cork on water it could suppose a 'will-to-float'. It exploited biology by spicing it with anthropomorphism.

Descartes' 'reflex action' performs, as he himself assigned it, a further rôle in our doing the things we do. Besides being complete robots in a number of our reactions to the outside world, we are still, he thought, in part robots when acting under 'reason' and 'will'. When these impel us, it is still the non-mentalized robot which executes what 'reason' and 'will' dictate. Reason and will initiate their acts, but the carrying out of these acts is an affair of the reflex machinery, or 'robot'. Here Descartes had travelled altogether beyond Fernel. For Fernel even the transfer of food by the stomach to the intestine, even the storage of bile by the gall-bladder, were attributable to mind immanent in those organs, parts of the soul pervading the body—and he was careful to say that that soul was the one soul. Descartes, on the other hand, declared that even our most mentalized acts are, as to their actual performance, the work of a robot mechanism.

To-day's knowledge teaches that every so-called 'voluntary' muscle with its nervous supply is a little 'reflex' system. Any act, of whatever provenance, which employs such a muscle cannot fail to enlist reflex action from it, and from muscles related to it—synergists, antagonists. These (proprioceptive) reflexes are unconscious as such, but on them depends in large part the rightness of the muscular act. They adjust duly the muscles' length and tension. They control duly its starting and its going out of action. This reflex factor is as important for the right performance of the movement and posture as is the tuning of a string for the harmonious use of it in music. This tuning is just part of the reflex robot operation of the body. We are not conscious of these reflexly maintained and adjusted muscular lengths and tensions as such. They self-regulate themselves unconsciously. All we are aware of is their outcome in our act. With each movement of head or neck or limb, whether passive or active, the pattern of the unconscious proprioceptive reflex changes. We are aware only of the movement or posture which is its accompaniment. Often even this latter is not within the field of our direct attention. Our attention is directed to the 'aim' of the act, not to the 'how' of it; the 'how' often enough takes care of itself. Conscious effort would seem unable to put us in touch actually with the proprioceptive reflex itself. So elusive is this last, that for long our muscles were unrecognized as affording any sensual basis of our motor acts. When we bend a finger we can, without looking at the finger and without the finger touching anything, tell within a little how much or how little we bend it; no hint, however, is vouchsafed to us that muscles doing the act lie up the forearm, or of the tensions or lengths they assume in doing it. When we turn our gaze we are not aware of the muscles of our eyeballs, nor can any mental effort or intensity of purpose make us so. None the less, the unconscious reflexes at work in them are indispensable to the due performance of our act. A critical incision by the surgeon, despite all his will and skill, could not be adequately done were these muscular reflexes, which unconsciously collaborate in it, to fail him.

Descartes' scheme thus makes this robot machinery of the muscles (proprioceptive) the servant of two masters. Anatomy diagrammatizes this. Graham Brown's cat or dog, retaining only its spinal cord and the immediate spinal annexes of the brain, is a reflex auto-maton. When placed on the moving platform it walks, runs, or gallops in agreement with the speed of the platform. The robot machinery of its limbs is started by the very movement communi-cated to them by the platform. This same reflex can be touched into just similar action by applying a feeble electric current to a point in the cross-face of the spinal cord close behind the head. The animal then starts walking, on strengthening the current its walking becomes running, and on further strengthening becomes galloping. The minutely limited stimulus has found a slender path of nerve-fibres coming from the brain (removed) which—diagrammatically stated —puts the brain's (conscious) action through to the unconscious robot in the spinal cord. The robot mechanism for walking is thus at command of (1) the external world, e.g. Graham Brown's plat-form, (2) the internal or cerebral or mental world, summed up by Descartes as 'reason' and 'will'. Shift the minute electric stimulus a little on the cross-face of the cord and stepping ceases. A nearby point can be found whence the limbs can be started doing something else, e.g. grooming the fur behind the ear, an act which can likewise be induced by rubbing the fur itself. Again, the robot is at the call of either world, the external (Fernel's macrocosm) or the internal (Fernel's microcosm) actuating the robot from the brain through the descending spinal path. The robot machinery is one and the same for both—namely, in this case, ultimately proprioceptive.

In evolutionary history, behaviour such as that part of our own which Descartes relegated to 'reason' and 'free-will', seems of later development than is the robot-behaviour, operated reflexly. The more primitive animals are less mentalized, and these, where there is a nervous system, manage to live mainly by 'reflex' action. Their quota of mentalized behaviour is relatively small, and in some instances vanishingly so. Descended from a long stock of less mentalized creatures as we are, and living less reflexly than did they, our more mentalized status has arrived at putting the reflex mechanism as a going concern, within the control, to a certain extent, of the reactions of the brain. This mastery of the brain over the reflex machinery does not take the form of intermeddling with reflex details; rather it dictates to a reflex mechanism 'you may act' or 'you may not act'. The detailed execution of the motor act is still in immediate charge of the reflex. Our individual history exemplifies this. A child late in 'learning to walk', which has perhaps never yet walked, will unexpectedly get up and walk passably well. Its walking has come to it as part of its growth; its mind simply had not earlier given it the cue. One of Shakespeare's characters exclaims, 'Mind is the slave of life'. That is profoundly so; but of all life's slaves, mind, though the most enlightened, is the most prone to truant.

It is largely the reflex element in the willed movement or posture which, by reason of its unconscious character, defeats our attempts to know the 'how' of the doing of even a willed act. Breathing, standing, walking, sitting, although innate, along with our growth, are apt, as movements, to suffer from defects in our ways of doing them. A chair unsuited to a child can quickly induce special and bad habits of sitting, and of breathing. In urbanized and industrialized communities bad habits in our motor acts are especially common. But verbal instruction as to how to correct wrong habits of move-ment and posture is very difficult. The scantiness of our sensory perception of how we do them makes it so. The faults tend to escape our direct observation and recognition. Of the proprioceptive re-flexes as such, whether of muscle or ear (vestibule), we are unconscious. We have no direct perception of the 'wash' of the labyrinthine fluid, or, indeed, of the existence of the labyrinths at all. In their case subjective projection, instead of indicating, blinds the place of their objective source. Correcting the movements carried out by our proprioceptive reflexes is something like trying to reset a machine, whose works are intangible, and the net output all we know of the running. Instruction in such an act has to fall back on other factors more accessible to sense; thus, in skating, to 'feeling' that edge of the skate-blade on which the movement bears. To watch another performer trying the movement can be helpful; or a looking-glass in which to watch ourselves trying it. The mirror can tell us often more than can the most painstaking attempt to 'introspect'. Mr Alexander has done a service[1] to the subject by insistently treating each act as involving the whole integrated individual, the whole psycho-physical man. To take a step is an affair, not of this or that limb solely, but of the total neuro-muscular activity of the moment—not least of the head and the neck.

Book VII, the last of Fernel's 'Physiology', is headed 'On the Procreation of Man'. Its preface says, 'now finally we have to enter

[1] *The Universal Constant in Living*, 8°, London, 1942.

upon "hidden and occult causes" and on much which is obscure and inexplicable'. Only a generation ago, Édouard Gley, in an address inaugurating the academic year in Paris, remarked that 'determinism', in the shape of physics and chemistry, was yearly triumphing more and more in biology, but that 'one theme there was which those sciences would never take over, the growth of the egg into a child'. To Fernel, four hundred years earlier, that theme may well have seemed, as his words say, 'hidden and occult'. We have already seen how he dealt with it in his 'Dialogue'. The 'Dialogue' enters into it at somewhat greater length than does the 'Physiology'. Factual knowledge about reproduction at the time of the Renaissance still remained scantier than might have been expected. Joubert's *Erreurs Populaires* bear witness to that. In the 'Dialogue',[1] Brutus, standing for the man of liberal culture of the time, declares that though the oak comes from the acorn and the bird from the egg, most things which arise and grow, such as metals, stones, seedless plants, animals traceable to putrefaction, spring *de novo*, without seeds. That the stones in the farmer's fields multiply is still a belief of our own country side.[2] Brutus, presently, adds to his list of the things which arise *de novo* without seeds, 'flies, snakes and mice'. Eudoxus opines that the sun accounts for this production. 'Snakes, locusts, worms, flies, mice, bats, moles, and all that sort of creature which, we incline to say, spring up *sua sponte* from rotting material draw life from the heavens.' And, as a gloss on that, he notes that the life-soul of the parent does not give rise to, is not the source of, the life-soul of the offspring.[3] Even where there are seeds, they cannot produce without the heavens.[4] Nothing is generated without the help of heaven.[5] This is conveyed in the Pythagorean saying of Virgil, *Omnia plena Jovis*. The procreation of man is effected not by man alone; the divine participates in it.[6] The 'form' is the life, and the heaven of stars, the eighth sphere, is a great reservoir of 'forms'. From that great source derives each and every human form—each new human life.[7] It comes by way of Sol, the planet. The 'Dialogue' tells us by the mouth of Eudoxus: 'Provident nature has given to the race of higher creatures, produced by the revolution of the stars, a reservoir of life, which is placed within the heavens that it may not die out.'[8] At the beginning

---

1 *Dialog.* i, c. 8. 2 Cf. B. Zincke, *A History of Wherstead*.
3 *Dialog.* i, c. 7. 4 *Ibid.* c. 8. 5 *Ibid.* c. 10.
6 *Ibid.* c. 7; also c. 10. 7 *Ibid.* cc. 7, 8. 8 *Ibid.* c. 8.

of the fourth month of pre-natal life, when the heart and brain are sufficiently advanced, there enters suddenly into the pre-natal child 'in a moment of time' the immortal soul.[1] 'Sol and man generate man', says the 'Dialogue'.[2] Between the account given in the 'Dialogue' and the shorter account in the 'Physiology' there is the difference that the planet Sol is not specifically referred to in the latter, evidence perhaps of Fernel's increasing caution as to astrology, the 'Dialogue', as mentioned above, being *written* earlier than the 'Physiology'.

The immortal soul suddenly entered the pre-natal child in the fourth month, but, owing to the plethora of the humours at that time, it remained in a state resembling drunkenness or torpor, unable to exercise its proper functions. At first, in this early period, the soul —and Fernel quotes Aristotle on this point—is 'animal' rather than 'human', and then specifically human, and finally it becomes individually human—'the soul of this man'.[3]

So ends this earliest treatise systematically setting forth human physiology as an integral subject. Fernel tells us his reason for writing it. 'Some when they have "done" anatomy and "done" their philosophy, straightway practise the art of healing. But that is to rush into a darkness, which their eyes will never pierce. Physiology tells the causes of the actions of the body.'[4] The subject had in its time, innovation as it was, to create a place for itself. It was doubtless helped toward that, by being first issued under the title 'On the Natural Part of Medicine', which equated it at once with a definite group of the studies of the Faculty. Its vogue must quickly have become considerable; it was printed three times in the next nine years. Then Fernel re-edited it, with but little alteration,[5] changing its title however to 'Physiology', a name by which the subject has been known ever since. His is the original introduction of the modern usage of the term. It was quickly adopted in Paris. Jacob Sylvius, Fernel's colleague, employs it in 1555,[6] that is, thirteen years after Fernel's first introduction of it, and only one year after Fernel's use of it as title for Part I of his *Medicina*. Not until some forty years

---

1 *Physiol.* vii, c. 13. 2 *Dialog.* i, c. 7, p. 76 and fig. 9, p. 40.
3 *Physiol.* vii, c. 13. 4 *Physiol.* ii, praefatio.
5 Note XIII, *Appendix*, p. 182.
6 *In Hippocratis et Galeni physiologiae partem anatomicam isagoge;* printed at Paris by I. Hulpeau, 2°.

later did the word in this new sense appear in English. A translation by 'A. M.' of Guillemeau's *Surgery* in 1597, says: 'Physiologia handleth and treateth of the structure and situation of Man's bodye.' In 1615 Crooke, in the *Body of Man*, has 'amongst the new writers Fernelius, the best learned of Physicians of them all, in the 7th book of his Physiologie', etc. A full-sized Commentary on Fernel's

IOAN. FERNELII
,Ambiani, Phyſiologiæ Lib. vij.

DE PARTIVM CORPORIS HVMANI
DESCRIPTIONE, LIBER PRIMVS.

10   Quo'doctrinæ atque demonſtrationis ordine ars medica con-
ſtituenda ſit,   Cap. I.

[decorated initial C] Vm liber ſolutúſque eſt animus, nudas & apertas rerum ſubſtátias perſpicuè cernés, clariſſima omnium cognitione fruitur: in hoc verò corporis velut ergaſtulum cóiectus, obrutúſq; obliuione tanquá deſa caligine, in ſumma verſatur ignoratione ſerum. At nihilominus ſemirta quædam etiamnū retinens diuinitatis ſuę,rerúmque maximarū dulci recordatione quaſi igniculis accenſus,perpetuo ſciendi noſcendique deſiderio flagrat. Hinc magno cum labore & ſtudio multa recuperat perſcrutatúrque ſenſuum ope, atque in ea primùm incumbens, quæ ſenſibus ſunt obuia, occultiora tandem ratione colligit ſola mente comprehenſa. Ita quidem à ſenſibus tanquam à certis rerum internunciis ſtabilita olim fuerunt diſciplinarū principia, è quibus demum perfecta omnis humana cognitio ducta deriuatáque eſt. Hæc ſumma eſt inueſtigandi faculeas,quam probatiſſinii quique l'hiloſophi ἀνάλυσιν, id eſt diſſolutionem appellarunt: quæ nimirum vel à toto & vniuerſo ad partes,& ſingula, vel à cópoſito ad ſimplicia, vel ab effectu ad cauſam, vel à poſterioribus ad priora ſerie deducens, abditiores illas cauſas inueſtigat, ex quibus ſingula ortu proceſſerunt. Huic aduerſa eſt altera componendi ratio, quam maximè natura nónunquam & ars ipſa ſequitur, ex partibus ea totum, ex ſimplicibus compoſitum, ex cauſis effectus, ex prioribus poſteriora nectit, atque id omnium primum ſtatuit, quod diſſoluendo poſtremum fuit perueſtigacum. Doctrinæ ſuæ initium ab analyſi duxerunt, quibus curę fuit omnia dilucidè atque,certo demóſtrationis nexu confirmare. Sic Geometriam & Arithmeticen Euclides,ſic Aſtronomiam Ptolemæus, ſic & Philoſophiam Ariſtoteles poſteris tradidit,eáque ſolida doctrinæ ſuæ fundamenta iecit, è quibus mulla tandem producerentur incredibilia vulgo & móſtri vel portenti ſimillima. Hos igitur quaſi veſtigiis odorati tradendæ medicinę initium ab humano corpore ducemus,quod & artis ſubiectú exiſtit,& omnium primum ſenſibus occurrit notiſſimum : à quo dein per minima quæque de-
                                                    a   ducti

Fig. 16. *Medicina* of 1554; the subtitle for *Physiologia*.

'Physiology' was begun by Riolan père, in Paris, 1574, and finished in 1579.[1] The 'Physiology' itself went through thirty-one posthumous reissues in the next hundred years. It remained textually unaltered. Fernel's supposition that physiology wanted integral treat-

1 *In Fernelium de Elementis*, Paris, and *Comment. in vi libros posteriores Fernelii*, apud Th. Brumennium, and we know further that both Riolan père and G. Capell gave public lectures on it.

ment had therefore been right. Ever since his own 'Physiology', treatises on physiology have continued to appear, onward to our own time. Fernel's retained its high place until the end of the seventeenth century. Then Boerhaave, the best known teacher of medicine of that time, advised that all physiological treatises written prior to Harvey's *De motu Sanguinis* [1628] were superannuated by this latter; Harvey's discoveries had given wholly new meanings to the heart and to the blood.

What impression does Fernel's treatise leave on us to-day? Unlike much of the medical writing of its time it is not prolix; it says what it has to say powerfully and clearly and closely. It has learning and originality; it drew to itself troops of readers, and it continued to have readers even after a hundred years. It contained some new observations. It set forth—admirably systematized, I would say—an up-to-date version of the then orthodox theory of the living of the healthy body. The titles of the consecutive books and chapters give in themselves a logical epitome of that doctrinal system. Running through all is an implication that the body is the scene of processes which, could our senses get at them, would supply medicine with its long-needed clues. It says too that dissection, useful though it is, will only indicate where the processes take place, not what the processes are—a point missed by Vesal. Observation of health and sickness was, to Fernel's thinking, the only way to learn what the processes are. Also he held, against the consensus of the Faculty, that the theory of medicine, as well as its practice, was not yet perfected—was still incomplete. The need was, he thought, for a supreme commentator, a 'conciliator', to reconcile the contradictions, and sift the statements, of the authoritative masters of the past. It was to that task, in no spirit of self-conceit, that he addressed himself when writing the *Medicina*, the first instalment of which was this 'Physiology'.

Fernel's presentation of his subject has certain negative merits. For its time it is relatively free from superstition. The Renaissance was superstition-ridden. Fernel was learned when to be learned was largely to be learned in superstition. His physiology eschews natural magic and is practically free from astrology. In these ways the pages of his book face hitherward.

But the book bears, plainly enough, stigmata of its time. It could not be otherwise. The circumstance makes it all the more interesting a document. Facts do not decay, and such new facts as the treatise brings forward are as much of to-day as of then. But it is different when we turn to its views on more general problems; there the book recedes into the past. Take that biological concept, which its time styled 'a faculty'. The immaterial tenant of the body, the life-soul, operated the body by means of faculties. Each main kind of action of the body bore witness to a 'faculty'. Thus, 'nutrition' was worked by a 'faculty', which had power to draw from the veins material renewing the flesh. Fernel observes that a child, while wasting with fever, may yet grow in stature. Therefore, he teaches, besides the nutritive faculty, there is a 'growth-faculty'. This resort to faculty-finding amounted sometimes to little more than the allotting of a name.[1] It was as though to name were to solve. Molière burlesqued this in the physician's tracing the sleep-producing power of opium to the drug being 'dormitive'. It was the old scholastic habit of *clocha clochabilis*, as Rabelais said.[2] Fernel did not wholly escape. In a satire of the time, written in dialogue, he appears for a moment and is asked 'what a "cause" really is'.[3] For Fernel in all earnest the living body had a principle *in* it but not *of* it. The body did not work itself. It was worked by an incorporeal principle within it. The healthy body did not undergo putrefaction because an immaterial life-soul, single and immanent throughout the whole, kept it alive in every part. In short, the body as body had not life. It owed its living to a spirit within. Fernel, disciple of Aristotle, was in this respect further from us in his sixteenth century of our era than the great master had been in his third century before our era. Aristotle conveys the impression of the body being its own prime-mover: 'There is however one peculiar inconsistency which we may note as marking this and many other psychological theories. They place the soul in the body and attach it to the body without trying in addition to determine the reason why, or the condition of the body under which such attachment is produced. This however would seem to be a real question calling for solution.'[4] For Fernel the tie between the various activities of the individual life is that they are so many 'faculties' of one immaterial life-soul, which latter is not of the same category as the body itself. For

1 'To tell us that every species of things is endow'd with an occult specific Quality, by which it acts and produces manifest effects, is to tell us nothing' (Isaac Newton).
2 Alphonse Lemerre's *Rabelais*, I, p. 19, Paris, 1879.
3 *Moyen de Parvenir*, de Verville.
4 *De Anima*, I. 3, §§ 22–3. Wallace's translation, p. 35.

Aristotle the tie between them all was that all were operations of the one and the same body itself. Fernel's view of the body, however, is not a merely static one like that of Vesalius—just a gross shape in frozen time.[1] The living body is expounded by Fernel as a dynamism, but it is a spirit-dynamism—so spiritist that it leaves little or nothing for chemistry and physics to do. To-day physiology *is* chemistry and physics.

What then of his treatise as an origin for the physiology which followed, and is following? It dates back less than four hundred years, and that is not long as human history counts time. Let us think. Its ingredients are the four humours, the three spiritus, the innate heat and the anima, or life-soul, with its various faculties. Of these the four 'humours' are, at least, 'matter'. But they are matter in the shape of the fictitious four elements which were not elements; and they, further, carry the fiction of the cardinal qualities of nature which were not cardinal. Then, the three 'spiritus'? These were a liaison between the matter of the body and the immaterial life-soul within it. The 'innate heat' was one remove further from matter. It derived from the quintessence of the heavenly sphere and from the stars. It reached the body by an occult ray, *via* the sun.

Coming to the 'faculties', we find them frankly spiritist; they are activities of the immaterial life-soul. Even had chemistry and physics existed there would, in Fernel's scheme, have been little place for them. But what a field for magic and astrology! To our surprise, Fernel forbids these latter almost wholly. Nature, he says, among his later writings, has laws, which hold good in the living body, even as outside it. Magic did not, he concluded, nowadays intermeddle in the body, whatever it might have done in times past. Toward the end of his life, in 1554, in the preface to the latest written part[2] of his *Medicina*, he wrote: 'Nothing whatever is discoverable in man which does not obey Nature and Nature's laws, save and except only man's understanding and man's free-will. Nature throughout is one eternal law, and Medicine is a book written within that law.' And so, in his 'Physiology', magic, transgressing that law and claiming to disregard that law, has for Fernel little place. We have only to turn to some of Fernel's contemporaries—to the distinguished

1 The admission however does not exclude the *De Fabrica* from a leading place in the biology of its century. Cf. Harvey Cushing, *A Bio-bibliography of Andreas Vesalius*, edit. J. F. Fulton, New York, 1943.
2 The 'Therapeutics'.

and liberal-minded Dean of Montpellier—to be faced by the difference between them. Fernel therefore, with all his errors, is yet an origin for the physiology of to-day. Truth emerges more readily from error than from confusion, wrote Francis Bacon. Fernel's 'Physiology' may be thought of as systematic error, but it is not confusion.

Physiology in the treatise of Fernel is an orderly logically constructed subject, so rounded-off that few loose ends remain to it, and hardly a growing-point. It is suspiciously complete. The four elements by their four qualities introduce the temperaments, the temperaments invite the humours, the coctions presuppose the organs, the organs require the spiritus, the innate heat demands the heart, the faculties consummate the occult, and are themselves consummated by—crowning concept—the 'life-soul', the *anima*. In result, that which was to be demonstrated is demonstrated, Q.E.D. Contrasted with this self-contained theorem, the physiology of to-day appears a thing of patches, ragged, untidy, fringed with loose ends, amorphous, confessing uncertainties, but, on the other hand, bristling with facts and growing-points. And, by comparison with Fernel's, how versed in Nature, how capable in daily life, how relatively effective in the sick room! The system which Fernel unfolded was logical but artificial, too humanly logical to resemble Nature. Fernel, proud of the Renaissance in which he moved, and of which he was an ornament, would have been pained to hear, that, as regards medicine, he and the Renaissance, with all their zest for doing and for progress, were still in reality little forwarder than were the Middle Ages. He who was to complete Medicine, the great commentator and conciliator, whose advent was looked for by Fernel, to clarify and recodify Medicine, did come, and in the shape of Fernel himself. Cabanis, in the late eighteenth century, wrote of Fernel that he was 'un génie capable de systématiser les connaissances de plus vastes'. An eighteenth-century hand has noted in Allbutt's copy (1680) of the *Medicina* 'Bordeu plaçait Fernel jusqu'à niveau avec Galen'. But far more were wanted than comment, conciliation and mere systematization. There had to be re-foundation. These four elements excogitated, but not known to experience. The four 'qualities', incapable of measurement, yet accepted as the whole fabric of health, nutrition, disease, and life and death—so intangible that there was still dispute which was the 'hotter', childhood or manhood.[1] Yet

---

1 Cf. Paparella, *op. cit.* ii, c. 15, fol. 42–3.

the spirit of the Renaissance was content with these things and endorsed the four qualities as established knowledge! They and the cardinal humours, the spiritus, the 'innate heat', the faculties, the life-soul, all of them overdue for liquidation. Their place would have to be taken by naked facts instead. The call was for wholesale demolition and wholesale reconstruction.

That long overdue change did at last begin. Re-foundation did start, but not in the age of the 'revival of letters', not in the age of the Renaissance; not until well on in the seventeenth century, the age of Descartes, Galileo and Gassendi. To carry it out was indeed beyond the power of one man, or of one generation; it demanded many men and many generations. It called for human co-operation the civilized world over.

It began, and is in active progress to-day. If the compunction lay on us, for convenience of retrospect, to attempt to identify some one particular event as the original step, our choice might fall on the discovery of the meaning of the blood and heart. The more so since it revived a method, as Sir Henry Dale has recently insisted, long disused—the coupling of observation with experiment. It was an innovation fertilizing medicine and science for a great harvest still ahead.

Part III

SUCCESS & THE CLOSE

WE PASS now, following the years, to Fernel's short treatise on blood-letting (Paris, 1545). It insists on moderation in that practice. Its prefatory letter is Fernel's nearest to vehemence in any of his writings. It addresses itself to all 'who practise Medicine, and hold it high'. 'The blood', it reminds readers, 'is the prime humour; to remove it in large quantity is to upset the very temperament itself. Withdrawal of blood is a most drastic remedy; yet it is done even in the enfeebled, yes, and in young children, as if loss of blood were a bagatelle; and the bleeding is repeated even three times, five times, and more.' In the next century Patin's letters [1] refer to a boy of seven who was bled thirteen times within a fortnight. 'The physician to-day', wrote Fernel, 'seems athirst for blood. Blood-letting, like wine-drinking, is right enough in moderation, but in excess it leads to disaster.' This small volume was soon reprinted—Lyons, Venice, 1548, and then again Lyons, Venice, 1549. It gave deep offence in the Faculty, and the vehement preface was omitted from a later edition.

A reader of to-day may feel some surprise to find this treatise discussing at considerable length what particular vein to open in affection of this or that organ or part. There was of course no suspicion of a general circulation of the blood. Parts above the collar-bone were said to be relieved by bleeding from the vein of the corresponding upper arm; parts below the collar-bone by the vein at the elbow. The blood-letting acted by an ill-understood process called 'derivation'. We still observe that to relieve ear-ache the leech must 'bite' near behind the ear. It is significant that in this tractate on blood-letting, with its details on the regimen and preparation of the patient, etc., and other precautions to be borne in mind, Fernel, in 1545, does not even mention the 'Egyptian days', or the 'critical days', or the mansions of the moon, or the sun or other planets. In his books of 1526 and 1527, though they were not wholly medical, he had dealt with these, and given a whole folio page and

1 *Lettres choisies de feu Mr G. Patin*, vol. 1, p. 8. Paris, 1692.

schema to the mansions of the moon. But in 1545, after stating
some commonsense rules about the preparation of the patient, he
adds, 'these rules are better than astrology'.[1] The tract was incorporated in the large systematic *Medicina* of 1554 as book ii of the
'Therapeutics', but shorn of the original preface.

Fernel's practice became very large. It left him scant time even for
his midday meal. His patients were of diverse rank, attendants at the
court, dignitaries, officials, visitors to Paris, and many of the poor.
He never neglected the poor. He had started poor himself; he died
a man of more than medium wealth. He was one to whom in his
profession money seems to have come plentifully without his
troubling greatly about it. Plancy, who lived with him, says he was
careful in the management of his house, but generous. On his
father withdrawing an allowance after a certain time, feeling the
other children must in their turn have the parental help, Fernel,
accepting the decision, had still persisted in his course, facing
penury. Later, in pursuit of astronomy, he had spent beyond
his means; and again later, when it was a question between a
remunerative practice and scantly paid teaching, he had, despite
advice of family and friends, held to his teaching. In the 'Therapeutics' (bk. iv, c. 6) we meet a significant remark: 'The "grain" is
the basis on which other weight-measures rest. Goldsmiths call it the
grain (lat. *momentum*) and it is constant and the same in all nations.
What preserves it unassailably, inalterably and without risk of super-
session is man's detestable thirst after gold, and his furious lust for
wealth.' Plancy tells us that, during the ten years he lived with
Fernel, his master rarely earned less than 'ten thousand pounds'
(*librarum gallicarum*) a year, and sometimes more than twelve thousand.
There is evidence that for the last accouchement of Catherine de
Medici (1556) he was paid 'two thousand three hundred Tournai
pounds'. Pierre Bayle gives an authority for stating that at Fernel's
death there were found in his study thirty thousand 'écus d'or'.[2]

After his tract on 'Bleeding', he gave such time as he could to
writing a system of medicine which he had long set his mind on
producing. He was never to complete it, but in 1554 he issued a
large instalment of it. It was made up of a republication of the
'Natural Part of Medicine', under the title 'Physiology', followed
by a new work entitled 'Pathology', and finally by a 'Therapeutics'

---

1 *De Vacuandi Ratione*, c. 13.   2 *Dictionn. Historique et Critique*, vol. II, 1697.

in three books, of which the second book was a reissue of the tract on 'Bleeding'.

The 'Pathology' became, in medicine, undoubtedly Fernel's best known work. Plancy remarks of it, and of the manner of its com-

IO. FERNELII

AMBIANI,

Medicina.

AD HENRICVM . II. GALLIARVM
REGEM CHRISTIANISSIMVM.

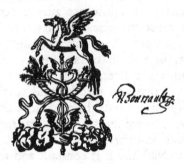

LVTETIÆ PARISIORVM,

APVD ANDREAM WECHELVM, SVB
PEGASO, IN VICO BELLOVACO.

1 5 5 4

Cum Priuilegio Regis.

Fig. 17. Fernel's *Medicina*, 1554; Andr. Wechel, son of Christ. Wechel, Paris, 2°.

position, 'in another few years he [Fernel] finished a distinctive and outstanding treatise on disease, and gave to it the name "Pathology"'.[1] He incorporated in it 'all that is good, and that stands confirmed on a solid basis, in the ancient masters, and added on his own part what his experience found they had omitted. He removed uncertainties, cleared up obscurities, corrected errors, and excised the superfluous.'[2] In fact he was here taking up, in the public interest, the

1 'Praeclarum atq. illustre de morbis opus cui pathologiae nomen indidit.'
2 *Vita.*

task which, as he saw it, was the greatest need of medicine, namely the digest of it by a trustworthy commentator and conciliator, a step towards 'codification'.

The 'Pathology' in several ways broke new ground. Not merely was the name new, but, as treated, the subject was new. It was not, as was then usual, a collection of 'cases',' a 'century' or 'bi-century' as commonly so-called. It was a systematic essay on morbidity, pursued unhaltingly through the body, organ by organ. Fernel is to-day sometimes mentioned as the 'father of Pathology'. He has some claim. At a time when the theory of medicine was still humoral he declared 'the fevers are of general and indeterminate seat in the body, but much disease has a special and localized seat in this or that organ'. He made this latter the basis of a classification of diseases. He had already in his 'Physiology' devoted a long chapter to the procedure for conducting a necropsy; he made necropsy, as far as he could, a routine practice for elucidating disease. 'He classified *localized* diseases as *simple* when confined to a part of a single organ, *compound* when affecting the whole organ, *complex* when affecting a set of organs. This was a new step at a time when the humoral doctrine taught that every complaint 'from disappointed love to measles' was a disorder of the humours. Professor Long says Fernel's 'Pathology' 'came too early in medical history to break with the teaching of humours, temperaments and vital spirits of the ancients; yet he developed a more rational general pathology than they, and wrote a special pathology which in its organization falls little short of being modern'.[1] We perceive the extent of the advance made by Fernel when we compare with his 'Pathology' a well-known book 'On some hidden causes of disease and cure' (1507)[2] by Antonio Benivieni, sometimes accredited as founder of pathological anatomy. Benivieni's work is just on the old lines, a collection of a hundred and eleven 'cases'. The novelty was at one time claimed for it that it collated post-mortem findings with symptoms noted during life, but in that Benivieni's work 'merely continues the tradition long established by the more elaborate of the *Consilia* of physicians of the two preceding centuries'.[3] Benivieni is not in fact so full or precise as are many of his predecessors. But, apart from that, Benivieni's slender volume is,

1 *History of Pathology*, by Esmond R. Long, 1928, p. 63.
2 *De Abditis Nonnullis ac Mirandis Morborum et Sanationum Causis*, Florence, the Junta; the work appeared posthumously, edited by a brother, Jerome.
3 Lynn Thorndike, *History of Magic and Experimental Science*, 1934, IV, p. 586.

by comparison with Fernel's 'Pathology', a random gathering without pretence to logical sequence; it often displays rank credulity.
Fernel's treatise belongs to a different order of knowledge. It is a
systematic setting forth of the facts then known in its subject. It is
an organized treatment of them, and sifts them critically. Its matter
is more concrete than is that of his 'Physiology': less reference is
made to 'spiritus' and 'faculties'. Its one excursion into the occult
is in discussing the causation of the plague-like diseases.[1] The
'Pathology' contains some noteworthy observations: for instance,
the earliest mention of ulcerative endocarditis.[2]

Much therefore in the same way as he had introduced the term
'physiology' into medicine, Fernel introduced the term 'pathology'
in its usual modern sense. The term is not found in the *text* of Guy
de Chauliac's *Chirurgie*, written 1363, but is given an important place,
with Fernel's meaning, in the commentary on the *Chirurgie* by Joubert,
twenty-two years after Fernel. Professor Long's *History of Pathology*
declares Fernel's 'Pathology' 'the first medical work to be called a text
of Pathology'.[3] The word has had currency in that sense ever since.
As to the strict scope, which, when introducing it, Fernel intended
the word to have, a clue is afforded by his—doubtless following
Galen—choosing at first the word 'aetiology'[4] (1542) and then substituting 'pathology' for it (1554). Illustrating the same line of
thought in him, the treatise itself insists 'it is not enough to observe
diseases, we must also observe the causes of them'.[5] Castellus, in
Messina's *Lexicon Medicum* (1598), says under αἰτιολογία, 'some call
this "pathology"'. That which Fernel had in mind under 'pathology'
would seem indeed to be everything which is an efficient cause, in
Aristotle's sense, of the sick state. For instance, an obstruction, a
phlegmon, a tumour, inasmuch as these all were immediate causes
of the symptoms of the patient's illness. Morbid anatomy in this
way came under 'pathology', and so also did 'symptoms', as being
signs of immediate causes. Pathology, in the meaning of Fernel, was
therefore not exactly in scope the pathology of to-day. Medicine,
like an organism, grows, and, growing, subdivides and buds. Fernel,

1 *Pathol.* i, c. 7; to be contrasted with his account of their causation in the 'Dialogue', ii, cc. 11, 12, 13.
2 *Medicina*, v, 12, p. 159, 1554. For an (?) *appendicitis* see *Univ. Medicina*, path.
vi, 9, p. 303, 1567. And *infra* Note XVII, *Appendix*, p. 184.
3 *History of Pathology*, 1928.   4 *De Nat. parte Medic.* praefatio, 1542.
5 *Pathol.* i, c. 11.

separating medicine into three parts and calling one of them 'pathology', saw in 'pathologia' not any study ancillary to medicine but an essential part of medicine itself. In later times 'pathology' began to be identified more exclusively with morbid anatomy. Microscopy, developing, reinforced that tendency by making morbid anatomy more complete. With Fernel, however, 'pathology' was not purely anatomical. It stood for the causes of symptoms of the morbid process. He was early followed in this: thus, in 1578,[1] by Laurent Joubert, who says, 'pathology, that is, causes of the malady or symptoms'. The English translation (1591) of Guillemeau has 'pathologie treateth of the causes and occasions of the sicknesses'. The 'pathology' of Cohnheim, considered novel in the later nineteenth century, was less a new departure than a return to the idea of Fernel, always with the difference that in the meanwhile there had arisen the 'experimental method'.

The 'Physiology' and 'Pathology' of Fernel were, in each respective subject, the earliest systematic treatises. They both of them established their respective subjects under those names. Both were the product of the same mind and hand. It argues for Fernel a certain largeness and an originality of view. For such a step medicine had had to wait many centuries. Doubtless both subjects, as scattered fractions of medicine, had long been unobtrusively shaping, but it was Fernel who recognized that they wanted dealing with as integers; and he established them as such. And each of his two treatises won for itself a long individual run of active life. Even in the eighteenth century Boerhaave,[2] leading teacher of the time, still recommended Fernel's 'Pathology' as the best. As Part II of Fernel's *Medicina*, and then of the *Universa Medicina*, the 'Pathology' was reissued thirty-six times in little over a century, and it was obtainable as a separate volume even so early as the year following its first issue. Guy Patin, Dean of the Paris Faculty, in a letter of 1660, names it, then a century old, as the treatise in use in Paris. There were two-volume and three-volume editions of the 'Universal Medicine', and the separate volumes, it seems clear, could be obtained separately, though they were not published as nominally separate. The frequency with which successive parts come separately into the antiquarian book market to-day, and exist separately in old libraries, supports their

1 *La Grande Chirurgie*, Tournon, 1578; *Annotations*.
2 Note XIV, *Appendix*, p. 183.

being originally obtainable separately. The 'Pathology' clearly was especially in demand. But it was not until 1638 that it was published wholly independently, and in 1650 in French.

All the works of Fernel were originally in latin, even to the little volume of 'Consultations' published posthumously. No vernacular version of any of them appeared for close upon a century—with one exception, the seventh book of the 'Pathology'. This was translated into french and issued as early as 1579 in Paris. The same excerpt from him had been englished even earlier, 1575, by William Clowes, afterwards surgeon to Queen Elizabeth. Now the seventh book is that part of the 'Pathology' which deals with 'External Diseases', and its issue in the vernacular was for the sake of the surgeons. In England the surgeons and the barbers had come to terms with each other, and had amalgamated under Henry VIII in 1540. Their 'Commonalty' exercised their calling fairly amicably with, though customarily as subordinates to, the physicians. There was no university in London, but the College of Physicians was established there by Wolsey (Linacre) 1518. The King confirmed the 'Privileges' of the barber-surgeons in 1543. Galen was both physician and surgeon. But time divorced the two callings. There was strife between them, especially in Paris. There were in Paris two bodies of surgeons. One held their meetings in the Church of St Côme and were known as surgeons simply; the other in the Church of St Sepulchre, and were known as barber-surgeons. The two did not combine until 1656, when, each retaining its own rules, they became the 'Community of the Master Barber-Surgeons of St Côme'. The isolated publication in french of the seventh book of Fernel's 'Pathology' in Paris was an incident in a long-continued struggle engaging the Faculty and these surgeons of both kinds.

The Faculty (of Medicine) opposed the surgeons reading latin— or indeed their reading much at all. The quarrel was interminable. This same reason operated a century later to bring about the separate publication not only of book vii but of the whole of Fernel's 'Pathology', and in french. The surgeons were under, but not of, the Faculty.

The surgeon's ignorance of latin was held to debar him from professional and social equality with the physician.[1] His lack of

1 Cf. Riolan père, *Ad impudentiam quorumdam chirurgorum qui medicis aequari et chirurgiam publice profiteri volunt, pro veteri dignitate medicinae apologia philosophica*, Paris, 1577, 8°, D. Vallensem.

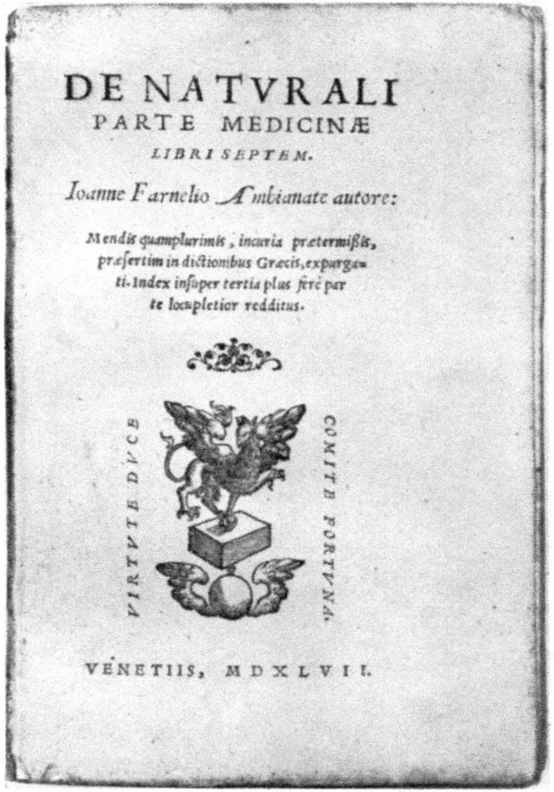

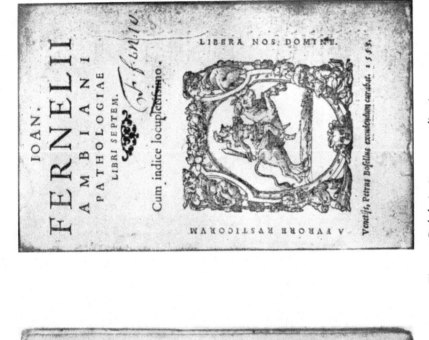

Fig. 18. *De Naturali Parte Medicinae*, 8°, Venice, 1547.

Fig. 19. *Pathologia*, 8°, 1555, earliest issue as a separate volume.

latin was often traceable to straitened home circumstances which could not afford the requisite schooling, or meet the expense of University. The preface to Dusseau's french 'Manual for Apothecaries' (1561) says it is written in french in order to help those apprentices—'tyroncles'—the poverty of whose parents has precluded their boys from learning latin.[1] This lack of latin in the surgeon prevented his direct access to the writings which physicians, and all the world, regarded as sources of authority for the art of healing. Also it cut him off from humane letters in an age which had come to attach transcendent value to them. Moreover, that he did not know latin was tantamount to a declaration that he was not a member of the Faculty of the University, and had never been at a College in the University, for at the Colleges in Paris in Fernel's day a fine was imposed for not speaking latin during meal times. Fernel's contemporary, the king's surgeon, Ambroise Paré, is said to have known no latin. Certain it is that, complete antithesis to Fernel, he wrote always in the vernacular.

The conflict between the physicians and surgeons in Paris was tripartite—a triangular duel. On one side the physician-doctors and doctor-regents of the University Faculty; on a second the master-surgeons of the College of Surgeons (the Collège de St Côme), founded[2] as far back as the early fourteenth century, under Philip the Fair, a College to which Lanfranc had somewhat later been attached. Ancient and of royal privilege though it was, the Collège de St Côme was outside the Faculties of the University. It could not confer degrees, doctor, master, or bachelor. But its members had the right to wear 'the long robe', and generation after generation strove to acquire a standing on equality with that of the doctor-physician of the University Faculty. They had a scutcheon resembling that of the doctor-physicians and they wore a four-cornered cap like that of the doctor of medicine. In 1544 they obtained from the king a privilege granting their enrolment of grammarian-clerks as pupils, knowing latin for the purpose of holding examinations in latin—the privilege expressly stating that it was to remove a disability and to bring the standing of the surgeons up to University rank. That the surgeons of St Côme did not customarily employ

1 *Enchirid ou Manipul des Miropoles*, traduit et commenté par M. Michel Dusseau, jadis Garde juré de l'Apothicairerie de Paris, pour les inérudits et tyroncles dudit estat, Lyon, Jan de Tournes, 1561, p. 40.
2 Under Philippe le Bel, by Edict, 1311. Cf. Quesney, *Hist. de la Chirurgie*, 1749.

latin for their lectures or proceedings seems clear from a report issued by the Dean of Medicine in 1506. The report describes a reception by the University Faculty in that year, held to hear from the Provost and Masters of St Côme a solemn affirmation of loyalty and obedience to the Faculty. The dean's account uses latin throughout, except for the affirmation by the surgeons and the question addressed to them, the only two items in french in the whole document.[1] The episode reads to-day like a victory for the Medical Faculty; the surgeons are described by the Faculty merely as adherents, 'scholars and disciples', of the Faculty, and not as having any definite rank either in the Faculty or University. Nevertheless, we find the surgeons of St Côme bringing it forward a hundred years later, as evidence in their favour in the old quarrel with the Faculty of Medicine—evidence that they are within the Faculty and members of it. How bitter the feeling was still in the seventeenth century is to be read in the letters of Guy Patin, then Dean of the Faculty of Medicine. He often reverts to it. The surgeons are 'booted lackeys... who wear moustaches and flourish razors'. Finally, the third party in the struggle consisted of the 'Corporation' of the Master Barber-Surgeons. In Fernel's time the great surgeon of the Renaissance, Ambroise Paré, the king's surgeon, was from the ranks of the Master Barber-Surgeons.

The status of the barber-surgeon was improving both in England and in France. But, for the earnest young surgeon, both in Paris and Montpellier, wanting his share of the best that was written in his subject, and not conversant with latin, there was very little to be found in the vernacular. On the other hand, every doctor of medicine, with his knowledge of latin, had the classics of surgery, such as Paulus Ægineta, open before him, and they were touched on as a minor part of his studies. But the false idea prevailed that manual operation being handicraft—which is indeed the literal meaning of the word 'chirurgy'—as such it was below the dignity of the learned. There was also the barrier which had been set up artificially by decisions of the twelfth- and thirteenth-century Church Councils. The art of healing had, in early Christendom, been an accepted preoccupation of the religious calling. But the express official declaration that the Church abhorred all shedding of blood (*Ecclesia abhorret a sanguine*)

---

1 Their lectures were in french in 1709; Le Verduc's *Maistre en Chirurgie*, Liège, 1709.

was taken to apply even to the medicinal letting of blood. Later, at the end of the thirteenth century, there was issued the injunction, from Honorius IV, which inhibited priest and monk from the exercise of medicine. Nevertheless, the overlap between the two callings long persisted. Linacre, physician to Henry VII, held three livings.

In the fourteenth century the confraternity of surgeons of St Côme sprang up in Paris, outside the Faculty of Medicine. It was the germ of the later College of Surgery in Paris. It had royal support. Our own Henry V and Henry VI, as kings of France, confirmed its privileges 'in letters tied with silk thread and sealed with green wax'. Successive kings of France confirmed them. Fernel's Henri II, on his accession to the throne in 1547, confirmed them. Fernel's pronouncement on the fundamental similarity and equality of surgery and medicine appeared seven years later, in his *Medicina* of 1554. It may well have seemed to some of his colleagues a disloyalty to the Faculty of Medicine. The development of a College of Surgery in Paris led to further rivalry between the Faculty and itself. 'Parlement' enacted that each surgeon must keep an open shop. The Faculty instituted a course in Anatomy based on 'Gui'—so de Chauliac was commonly styled—in latin with explanations in french, a physician to preside, a surgeon to dissect.

Montpellier was more liberal in its policy toward surgical education than was Paris. This was partly due, in his time, to the famous Chancellor of Montpellier, Laurent Joubert, Professor and Dean, and author of that 'best seller' of its day (Jan. 1, 1578), the *Erreurs Populaires*. He tried to straighten things out for surgery. We find him writing:[1] 'To our distress Surgery, the most ancient part of medicine, and the most excellent of all in respect of the results it has to show, is lamentably relegated to the hands of the artisan and simpleton.[2] It would have been even worse had not 200 years ago that worthy man, Guy de Chauliac, taking account of surgery's misfortune, carefully gathered up all that was best in ancient authority, and, a Herculean labour, cleansed true surgical art from the crudities

1 Letter to Catherine de Genas, 1 August 1578, p. 22, from *La Grande Chirurgie de M. Guy de Chauliac, etc.* composée 1363, restituée par M. Laurent Joubert, Lyon, 1580, 8°, pp. 713.

2 Cf. the preamble to the statute of Henry VIII dealing with a similar situation, in England, p. 23, *supra*.

and beastlinesses which disgraced it. A thousand superstitions had entered it, and magic, sorcery, trickery, cant and fraud, with endless errors and farce.'

So it was that Joubert undertook (Aug. 15, 1578) the fundamental re-editing of Guy's bicentenarian text. Besides dealing with the latin he issued a fresh french version, and his publisher, he tells us, insisted on the latter appearing at once, feeling it no doubt the more urgent of the two. There was already a french version in use, but 'so scabrous, gross, barbarous, difficult and obscure', Joubert says, that it had to be wholly recast. The terms in which the remark is couched are characteristic. Laurent was always loquaciously himself.[1] At intervals along the margins of his *Guy restitué* appears the astronomical sign for Jupiter, the planet. His foreword explains this[2]. 'I have indicated my annotations, where they occur, by the character ♃, which I have long employed as my personal device and symbol. The astrologers signify by ♃ Jupiter, and likewise, turning it upside down, Saturn. But right-side-up it spells the initial capitals of my name and surname, and I like it especially. Moreover, these same Jupiter and Saturn, son and father, were—so I understand—favourable at my birth. I have not been sparing of myself in making my annotations ample. I have done so for the sake of the young surgeons, who often have not the means for an education at our good universities, and have not the luck to meet first-rate scholars, so that they must pick up what learning they can through their own hard work and private study.' Laurent's son, Isaac, also of Montpellier, issued during his father's lifetime the latter's 'annotations' to Guy put into french.[3] He prefaces them by a statement which amounts to a contemporary gloss on the question of latinity and the surgeons. It is addressed to the President of the High Court of Dauphiné, to whom the whole volume is dedicated.

Sir, two years ago, I ventured 'a translation from latin into french of two of the *Paradoxes*[4] of M. Laurent Joubert, my honoured father and your attached servant. I have now made bold to go farther, and have

1 Haller called L. Joubert's diction 'Boccaciana & jocularis'.
2 *La Grande Chirurgie*, etc., Tournon, p. 10, in the 3rd edition, 1598.
3 *Annotations de M. Laurent Joubert, sur toute la Chirurgie de M. Guy de de* (sic) *Chauliac, etc.*, Tournon, 1598, 8°, pp. 403; Claude Michel, printer to the University. Isaac refers to his father who died in 1583 as then alive; hence a prior edition.
4 The *Paradoxes* were of 1561; the translation at least as early as 1580. *V. infra*, Note XVIII, *Appendix*, p. 185.

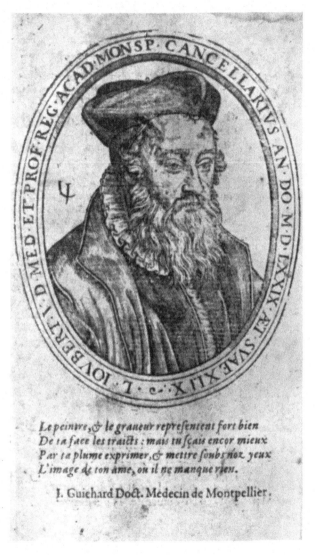

Fig. 20. Portrait of Laurent Joubert from *La Grande Chirurgie de M. Gui de Chauliac, restituée par M. Laurent Joubert*, Tournon, 1598.

translated into French his 'Annotations' on the surgery of M. Guy, for they are greatly in request. This I have done as much to save him trouble as to perfect myself further in the subject....I will deal here merely with the objections constantly urged against his translating the Surgery of Guy....It is physicians and surgeons especially who blame him. But they do so for quite different reasons. The physicians, honouring my father (and many of them have been his pupils and are famous in various parts of France), have said that for him to translate out of latin into french a book on surgery was an act unworthy of him, the more so seeing it was a book which can hardly be said to have an author, a mere collection and 'omnium gatherum' of bits from all and sundry written on surgery in old times and our own. For, say they, M. Joubert, famed for his learning in every University of Europe, should rather have issued the fruits of his own mind, original work of his own. Or, if he were bent on making better understood the thoughts of others, could have done so in ways more worthy of his repute, by translating works of the ancient masters, greek and latin, the great Fathers of Medicine, and by illuminating them with a commentary. But he must needs go to work on a Guy de Chauliac, a frequenter of the barbers' shops. What! a Chancellor, and Dean, and Doctor-Regent and Regius Professor of the foremost University of Medicine in the world, amuse himself with translating into french and penning commentaries on the fly-blown refuse of an old-time crank whom even most surgeons now disown, contemn and disdain! Could the Dean not at least have spent his time on translation from greek into latin, and, for instance, composing a copious commentary on the books of Hippocras, Galen, Paulus Ægineta and other good authorities? Could he not at least, as does M. Dalechamps, one of the best and wisest heads in France, render into french from the greek the 6th book of Paulus Ægineta, which treats of surgery, and comment on it? So it is they speak.

Let me at once answer the last point. My father had in fact that intention, and has several times in his lectures interpreted the 6th book of Paulus to the 'student-companions' in surgery as his audience. And because that did not thoroughly satisfy him, he translated the text afresh from the greek into french, and dictated it to the pupils. But after M. Dalechamps had published[1] his, he left the matter there and turned to the surgery of Guy.[2] Nor was he singular in this choice; he was confirmed in it by M. Gabriel Fallopius of Padua, and M. Jean Tagault[3] of Paris and M. the reverend Falco, formerly Dean in Montpellier. My father is

1 *Chirurgie francoise recueillie*, Lyons, 1570.
2 J. Canappe, 'reader to the surgeons of Lyons' issued a french *Commentaire* on Gui de Chauliac, Lyons, 1532.
3 Furnished a précis of de Chauliac's *Chirurgia Magna*, under title *De chirurgica institutione, libri 5*, Paris, 1543, 2°.

thus with them in wishing to honour the writings of this worthy doctor, a predecessor of himself in this our University, and in his time famed for rare knowledge and great experience in both medicine and surgery, not being in fact M. Guy a simple surgeon, or a common barber, as some think. They who think so are ill-informed as to his titles and quality. And, please God, may those who despise him come to understand him. That his language is uncouth is no reason for rejecting his doctrine; it is only one reason the more for translating it into better....

I come now to the surgeons. They are of two sorts, the one 'Latins', the other 'French'. We call 'Latins' the surgeons who have had the good fortune to be brought up 'literate', and to know latin and how to latinize. These are they who for the most part despise the work of Guy. They hold solely by the writings of Hippocras and other ancient authors. Or, if they sometimes read the surgery of Guy, they do so secretly as something to be ashamed of; nor do they acknowledge it as the source of what they get from it. And that is meanness and ingratitude—to deny acknowledgement to that from which one profits. Well, these surgeons are to be put in the same class with the physicians who despise M. Guy.

I pass to the other sort, who value this surgery highly, and yet protest against its being put into french, because in that way it becomes open to those who are ignorant of latin. They complain that it is improper for the mysteries and secrets of so excellent an art to be made known to mere barbers, some of them unable to read or write. But, as for these last, I say, it is all one in what language the book is, for they can read none. I grant it is very ill that the exercising of surgery, which I have heard my father call one of the worthiest parts of medicine, should be committed to ignorant illiterates (analphabetes) unable even to read. All they have is a certain routine, and some prescriptions learned by rote. Empirics they are, wholly innocent of any science. It amounts to a blasphemy.

But, on the other hand, there are those whose misfortune it is to have had neither kith nor friends able to support them at schools of grammar or letters, although they can read well enough, and are intelligent and studious, and love surgery. Why should all the treasure of learning in their subject, contained in latin and greek, be kept from them for want of translation into french? Talents are the gift of God. This man has the gift of languages, that of ingenuity, this is by nature an observer, that a born describer, one operates deftly and neatly, another excels in memorizing, another in power of inventing, yet another has some other talent, and all can contribute worthily to some calling and further the public good. But out of fifty of them there will not be perhaps two who understand latin. Must they all then be put off from surgery though brought up to it, bred in it, and wishful to learn it well, and to perfect themselves in it by means of good books, but perforce books in the everyday tongue? I conceive that some of the best and most competent surgeons of our time know no latin.[1] But I know they discourse and reason and discuss and consult excellently in french.

If it be objected that this will make them despise scholarship, and smile at those who would devote themselves to latin, and should it be argued further that, books in french being withheld, many of these non-latinists would, to the advantage of everyone, throw up the old career of their fore-bears which was a mistake for them, I reply that some of them have especial aptitude for the science and art of surgery in spite of not having had the wherewithal for lessons in latin when young. These, with a natural bent for the surgeon's calling, when they come under good instructors, can, if they have access to good books (which are silent instructors) arrive at great skill and knowledge. Would it not be a thousand pities if, for lack of the books, students such as these remained ignorant of their art, and mere empirics? It is not everyone, says the old proverb, who can get to Corinth. Nor does God dispense to all to whom he gives natural good sense—which is the half of knowledge—the means of linguistic study. There may be good judgment, good invention, industry, ability, refine-ment and liking for surgery; everything but latin! Then too, if the books which are read to these prentices in surgery are interpreted for them in french, and their disputation exercises are in french, why not allow them to have in french all they want to know. Books now-a-days carry further than public lectures, nor can all afford to attend lectures. Worthy Cato said, 'diffuse the teaching of anything good; do not confine it'.

But now I hear a remark from the latinist surgeons. They agree that books in our vulgar tongue are needed by those I mention. But, they object, for ten who will profit by them, a thousand will abuse the privilege. Besides those few who, in Minerva's despite, have taken up the profession, there are a crowd, they remind us, who, not actually of the profession, yet dabble in it. This mob, if prescriptions are published in the simple tongue, will take them and trade in them....But, I answer, abuse of good things is no reason for forbidding them altogether. How pitiful to grumble, and say, nothing about surgery shall be published in french, lest the means of treatment (the 'secrets') become public property and everybody employ them. Wicked, I say, and accursed, is he who rages and storms against the poor barbers, in their ignorance of latin, getting the facts which benefit himself. I repeat, the said barbers can possess talents from God both great and rare, and with the aid of such can go far, if they are not stopped by a string of words in latin.[2]

Here, in a vein of humour like his father's, he pauses to tell (as coming from Henri Estienne, the humanist printer) how a barber

1 Ambroise Paré it is said. He signed his first book 'Maistre Barbier Chirurgien'.
2 Abridged.

in a prescription read 'sacrifier' for 'scarifier', with what consequences to the patient he does not add.

An impression left from Joubert is that learning latin meant in sixteenth-century France an expense which only the reasonably well-to-do could bear. This would go to show that Jean Fernel's parents—his father was a furrier and innkeeper in a country town—were well-to-do. Goulin, commenting on the 'Life' by Plancy, thinks Fernel was well enough equipped in latin when he went to the University to be excused 'grammar'.

Despite some liberal advocates, the struggle of the surgeon for literacy and recognition continued bitter. In Paris in the year 1600 the barber-surgeons were still asking the 'Collège à longue robe' to implement their recognition, as directed by a recent decree. Their document of request shows the extent of proficiency and knowledge which the barber-surgeon candidates could offer.

Request to the Royal College of Surgeons of the Long Robe, in this town and University of Paris, on behalf of the Corporation of the Barber-Surgeons of the said town, presented by ten barber-surgeons chosen as delegates, who supplicate, saying that by Decree of the Court of Parliament made the last day of May, 1600, between you Gentlemen on the one hand, and the Community of the above Barber-Surgeons on the other, it was ordained that no one could pass for a master Barber-Surgeon in the town of Paris except in the presence of two Representatives of your College, who would be present at all the examinations and exercises which are carried out for the aforesaid Mastership, in order to approve them or reject them according as they are worthy or unworthy of the aforesaid Mastership. Following on the above Decree the supplicants above-named have since its date been received for, and gone through, the exercises and examinations of the said Corporation of Surgeons, and done so in the presence of two of you Gentlemen, deputed to be present at those examinations, and have been examined in their presence as also in that of the Dean of the Faculty of Medicine, accompanied by two other physicians of the said Faculty and of several Master Barber-Surgeons, on all things which pertain to surgery; namely, at the first examination, on diseases both general and particular, and both theoretical and practical, pertaining to the said Art, to wit: abscesses, wounds, ulcers, fractures and dislocations. In the first week they have been examined on the first day, on the nature, composition and articulation of the bones; the second day on affections which occur in the said bones, which are fractures, dislocations and caries, and on the remedies proper for such cases, such as ties, apparatus and bandaging. In the second week they have made dissections and demonstrations both general and particular of a human body and its parts, and that for the space of eight days making two lessons a day, one on the nature of the parts and the other on the affections which occur in them, and have made the operations requisite for the cure of them, such as the application of the trepan to the head, all the kinds of sutures to the face, the opening of empyema, puncture in dropsy, gastric suture of the belly, the ligature of anal fistula, the amputation of a limb, and many other operations which would take too long to specify. In the third week they have opened all the veins and arteries bleedable in the human body, and applied cuppings, and leeches. In the fourth week they have been examined on the properties of simple remedies and the composition of them, in so far as concerns the cure of the aforesaid diseases, which is all that is done and can be done by the competence of a Surgeon; and they have been, as well as by the Physicians, received by the Surgeons deputed by yourselves, as by all the other Barber-Surgeons of the above City, and approved capable and fit for the exercise of the said Art both in this City of Paris and anywhere else. So that the above Supplicants would desire to-day to enter into your Society and College, and be received, and acquire and have the insignia of Surgeons like your own.

In view of this, Gentlemen, and seeing that the said applicants have not yet proceeded to that final act, which you, my aforesaid Masters, are wont to do, entering into the above-named Society and College, which you call the act honourable, which is all that remains for them to do in order to be received into it: may it please you in your good pleasure to receive the said Applicants and to perform the said act, and without charge; that by that deed, they be admitted and received by you into your aforesaid Society, and have the marks and insignia of Surgeons, in the same way as you possess them in your houses, and, this doing, are bounden to the honour and duty needful and required in every honourable Society, and to render you each and all every honour and service you would wish them to render you.

Signed *Jean Menard*, &c.

October 17th, 1600.

This liberal view-point in the Jouberts went along with a social standing, which had in it something of gentlehood and inherited leadership of the country-side. Laurent's stock were of the landed gentry of the Dauphiné, and his writings show him animated by a sort of patriarchal devotion to the welfare of its people. It was bred in him to think of them, low and high, as *his* people. His popular book tries to disabuse them of their misconceptions and superstitions about health and its safe keeping. The *Erreurs Populaires*, had an unprecedented vogue. It was reprinted ten times in six months (Wickersheimer)! Its first issue was dedicated to

Marguerite de Valois, Queen of Navarre, the 'reine Margot' of anecdote, and idol of Brantôme. Though Margot was not a prude, that dedication had to be withdrawn, because parts of it erred in too great freedom of expression. The book had a Rabelaisian redundance.

Laurent Joubert was a man of many parts, Professor, Dean, and finally Chancellor, of the University of Montpellier. He was an authority on wounds inflicted by the arquebus, i.e. firearms in general. He advocated spelling reform, and invented a system for it; but could get no publisher to adopt it. His essay 'On Laughter' was famous, and is perhaps still read. His pages present a quaint discursive learning and a fund of humour often touched with pathos. They have a background of generous good sense characteristically his own. Wickersheimer[1] says of him, 'he can perhaps be compared with the greatest writers of his age. To-day is too neglectful of him.' The *Erreurs Populaires* is a sort of *regimen sanitatis*,[2] enlivened by a discursive wit. The following is from a 'dedication' prefacing his *Guy's Surgery restored*. He was then forty-nine. Amoreux,[3] in 1816, recalls this dedication as 'une épître remarquable'.

Therefore it is to you, Madam and most honoured Mother mine, that this offering belongs, in token of the right you have in respect of me, you who have brought me into this world, that I may have the privilege to do such service to you as I may. But, even if that were not so, there are in you such qualities that the veriest 'stranger in the land' (as the saying runs) did he hear the excellence of your merits were straightway moved to dedicate such a work to you.

For you yourself have undertaken the care and nursing of the sick poor, and have tended those ills which bring them to the Surgeon. Their abscesses, their wounds, their burns, their places which will not heal. Who is there can have seen, or read of, remedy more certain and more wonderful than your salve for inflammation of the breast? and with it you have cured a multitude of poor women who were almost in despair with pain and inflammation. Your ointment for burns, how admirable an assuagement! The Gualtier linen you keep for old ulcers, what a blessing to them! And then, your 'wine of absinthe', in our french 'aloyne', which you at some time invented, and made all from herbs out of the garden, and with wine from your own grapes; how excellent

1 *Op. cit.* p. 632.
2 Cf. *Regimē Sanitatis Roberti Gropretii*, Denys Janot, Paris, 1540, 16°.
3 P. J. Amoreux, preface to the 1816 re-issue of Lussauld's *Apologie pour les Médecins*, 1663.

and what a stand-by it is. I say nothing of all your preserved extracts and your distilled waters, prepared for the sick poor and in the love of God. For the rich have wherewithal, which they can take to the apothecaries and buy with. But not so the poor.

These are good works. The physician in me finds nothing but praise for them. They are not like the enterprises of some—presumptious apothecaries, foolhardy barbers, and others—who practise all sorts of remedies against right and reason, and get themselves well paid, not only for their divers drugs, but for their misdoings, their trickeries and their impudence. You, in all truth, make good and approved remedies and give them in charity, just as you would buy from the apothecary to give away. And of a truth you, I can say, make it your mission to play the surgeon and the apothecary for the poor, as indeed did your forbears before you, living nobly on their lands as members of an ancient house. Yes, so indeed was the custom of your house, to have its own remedies, prepared by womanly hands, for dispensing in charity to the sick and needy. We read the same of lords and dames, princes and princesses, Kings and Queens, of olden times. They gave themselves—and in France to-day there are noble souls who do so—to finding out and compounding certain medicaments which continue on in favour, retaining the names of their original authors. There is Gentian, King of Illyria, there are Lysimachus and Alexander the Great, Kings of Macedonia, John, King of Mauretania, Sabor and Ginger, Kings of the Medes, Archilaus, King of Cappodocia, Agamemnon, the Argive King, Sabriel, King of Arabia, Hermes and Ptolemy Philadelphos, Kings of Egypt, all these invented remedies; and let me end with Mithridates, King of Pontus and of the twenty-two nations of the different tongues, for he it was who devised and brought to perfection the ancient composition named from him 'Mithridate', still universally approved and keeping his name high. Other recipes there are which have not so stood. Among salves which shall last, I do not doubt, are those of Madam Chevallière Joubert, for healing divers maladies of the breast. Their renown runs through all Dauphiné, and the Lyonnaise, and Provence and our whole country round, and so it will be always. For a good thing is durable, and flourishes from the green juice within it.

Madam, it is not flattery which bids me write this. Truth, love of honour, and the reverence I owe you, would have me proclaim your dignity, your worth, and your most excellent disposition; what though the inevitable shadow shall come at end. And of all the labours of my life I have chosen this one to dedicate to you. And how could I do better than dedicate this re-writing of an excellent surgery to a lady who gladly has made it her christian pleasure to tend, oftimes with her own hands, the sick poor, with their sores, in charity and piety unbounded.

And now you are near to eighty years of age, sound in all ways and well. You have been granted twenty children of a marriage, all fair and strong and without blot or blemish. And of your children's children there are already eighty, so that you are now mother and grandmother of a hundred children. Have you not indeed the blessing that God promises by the mouth of his kingly prophet David in the hundred and twenty-eighth psalm!

Laurent Joubert this first day of August 1578, at Montpellier in the house of his mother. [This good son was in fact to die earlier than the venerable mother whom he was thus addressing.]

The quarrel over latin and the surgeons long outlived the century of Fernel. Guy Patin's letters of the mid-seventeenth century are savagely violent against the surgeons. Witness to the other side is the french Preface to the french translation of Fernel's *Pathologia* in 1646.[1] The translator took the *Pathologia* of the *Medicina*, not that of the *Universa Medicina*. The latter's variations from the former seem unknown to the translator, who veils himself under the initials 'A. D. M., docteur de Médecine'. His 'declaration', following next after the title-page, reads:

If knowledge of disease pertained only to those gentlemen, whose honour confines them to the responsibility of giving advice, and compels them to decline that of actual operation, contenting themselves with discourse, in a language which renders them more an ornament than a necessity, there would then be no need to publish in our vulgar tongue the mysteries of the Art, which they hide under the same veil as that commonly reserved for all that is most sacred. But since these delicate advisers upon Nature are pleased to derogate all manual operation to those so fully occupied with things to do as to miss the studying of words, those advisers ought not, I say, to begrudge the supplying of theory to those often obliged to practise it without other counsel than their own wits. The conjunction of Fate and the time and the disease does not in every case allow of seeking advice before treatment. And it can be presumed that he who can apply the remedy is not wholly ignorant of what is wrong. Yet he will perform his task the better for knowing the reason why. The author of this work [i.e. Fernel] is well-known.[2] Its matter is weighty. As to the style and manner of my version of it, I offer no excuses. If I am clear, that suffices me. No one can blame me for having done what within me lay for him for whom I undertook it. He can be grateful to me if he will. His gratitude is no affair of mine, any more than is approval

1 The only two copies known to me say 'finished printing in 1646' but have on the title-page 1650. Guy Patin's separate issue of the work in latin had been in 1638.
2 In the eighteenth century his name among surgeons was still one to conjure with: cf. Le Verduc's *Maistre de Chirurgie*, 3rd edit.

by the severely critical. Their censure will not move me so much as shall their charity.

Finally the College let the barbers join it. The Faculty went to law. The law deprived the surgeons of all Faculty rights; the term 'College' was forbidden to them. 'St Luke is stronger than St Côme', wrote Patin.[1]

That the surgeons' choice of a book to have in french should fall on Fernel's *Pathologia* was significant and natural enough. It was unequalled in reputation and its author's Preface contained a just tribute to surgery, which had doubtless, when it appeared,[2] embarrassed and annoyed the Faculty in Paris. The Preface said: 'Surgery is one with medicine. It rests on the same principles. In the development of those principles it follows the same essential ideas as does medicine.' Such a statement could at that time be twisted by the unscrupulous into a disloyalty to the Faculty.

In the *Medicina* of 1554 the third and final part was the 'Therapeutics', consisting however of three books only, the second the short treatise of 1545 on venesection and purgation. These latter subjects were coupled because both aimed at changing the humours. In the posthumous 'Universal Medicine' (*Universa Medicina*) of 1567, issued by Fernel's literary executor Plancy, the 'Therapeutics', completed from a MS. of Fernel, had four additional books, making seven. The 'Therapeutics' opens with a noteworthy preface, in which Fernel states finally his view of the relation of medicine to Nature. This preface prepares us for the exclusion of natural magic and astrology from therapeutics, and we find them in fact largely excluded. Fernel's preface tells us that Nature's laws are inviolable, even by the supernatural. Medicine comes under the dispensation of Nature. The laws of Nature obtain even within the body of man. It is Fernel's merit to take up this position in the mid-sixteenth century, a time when our own Linacre, the foremost humanist physician of his time, subscribed to magical treatment by sending twenty finger-rings, blessed by the king, to Paris as cures for rheumatism.

A key to Fernel's therapeutics is the doctrine of contraries—and he supplies a succinct statement of it.[3] The world is the scene of change and movement, and every kind of change and movement proceeds from the conflict between, and repulsion of, contraries. Nature stirs the world into continual action by sowing it everywhere with

1 10 fevrier, 1660.   2 1554.   3 'Therapeutics', bk. iv; preface.

antagonisms. As with the four elements, fire, water, air and earth, so with everything created, Nature opposes each by something else, its contrary. We may be sure there is no malady but Nature has made something contrary to it, and that contrary can remedy it. But we notice that Fernel's remedies, ransacking the world though he does, only meagrely include metallic and alchemical products. Fernel held that the benevolence of the Creator placed amongst the herbs of each country some which were the natural remedies for the diseases existent there. We have, he thought, only to find out which those herbs are. Though, even when found, it will still require long experience with them to know how to use them successfully. Exploration of that kind engaged him at the time of his death. In his last illness he prescribed eagerly for his own case, consulting frequently with colleagues.

As to his *armentarium*, we find (bk. vii) in it recipes which could claim to have been of repute for more than a thousand years. It is the reverse to-day when the antiquated remedy is rightly suspected of being out of date. Two venerable items in Fernel's list were the 'mithridate'[1] which we heard Laurent Joubert mention in his letter to Madam his mother, and 'theriac' which can be thought of as a modified 'mithridate'. The humoral theory ranked them as 'humid antidotes'. They were recommended for certain forms of pestilence and epidemic, and especially they were efficacious against venoms. 'Mithridates, like King Attalus, in Galen's native land, tested the effects of various drugs upon condemned criminals, and had discovered antidotes against spiders, scorpions, sea-hares, aconite and other poisons. He had then combined these into one grand compound which should be an antidote against any and every poison. He did not include in it the viper; this was added by Andromachus, chief physician to Nero.'[2] 'Andromachus then wished the name changed from Mithridate to Theriac because of adding vipers, to which he attributed the name θηρίον, and he made them the chief

<hr/>

1 Martial's *Epigr.* v, 76:
> Profecit poto Mithridates saepe veneno
> Toxica ne possunt saeva nocere sibi.

Rendered by W. T. Webb (*Trans. from Martial*, London, 1879):
> 'Drug-proof old Mithridates grew
> By frequent poisonous potation.'

Cf. also A. E. Housman's *A Shropshire Lad*.
2 Lynn Thorndike, *History of Magic and Experimental Science*, i, p. 170.

ingredient of the compound.'[1] Galen says theriac became almost the
food of his imperial patient, Marcus Aurelius. Fernel's 'mithridate'
contained fifty ingredients. Fernel and Plancy mention the Andromachus variant of the recipe. Plancy's annotation adds that there are
extant four forms of the original mithridate. Saguyer,[2] in his
lengthier commentary on Fernel's prescriptions, considers theriac
more efficacious than mithridate, but more acrid and less easily taken.

Looking through the prescriptions of the 'Therapeutics', not for-
getting the long history of ingenuity which had gone to their making,
constituent by constituent, each with a *raison d'être* behind it, we
appreciate Fernel's sympathy with the wish of Euripides that things
might have speech and tell us what they are. In these multiple
'poly-alexines' each ingredient had its place by right of its nature and
its share of the four cardinal qualities. Each brought a temperament
to the summed temperament of the whole. The complex was no
haphazard mixture. Its construction followed a sort of scholastic
logic, employing beliefs dating from Alexandrian and pre-Alexandrian
tradition. The physician was out to compass a total 'contrary' to meet
all aspects of the mischief suspected in the sick patient. The constituents
were chosen to support each other. Each item would lay claim to
being decisive of life or death given a certain conjunction of fate and
time and place. Fernel would have been amazed at the daring sim-
plicity, the impudent self-sufficiency of the remedies of to-day—their
directness, their specificity, their inequivocality. Substances, often
manufactured designedly by laboratory art, each entrusted single-
handed with subduing this or that otherwise intractable illness—
rickets, scurvy, pernicious anaemia, beri-beri, myxoedema, etc.[3] The
fatality of diabetes controlled by a single-substance extract. The
surgeon before operating precluding pain from the sufferer by ad-
ministering a little of this or that single definite and particular
chemical thing. Fernel had chafed against empiricism all his life, but
had seen it succeed where theory did not. But now he would find
us in a time when fuller knowledge is putting a groping empiricism
out of date. He would perceive that a new order of knowledge and
certainty has arisen for the art of healing. For himself and those with
and before him, uncertainty invalidated the very 'facts' on which

1 Chares, *L'Histoire des animaux de qui entrent dans la Thériaque*, Paris, 1668.
2 Cf. Bibliog. No. 124.U.
3 Cf. Sir Henry Dale, *Brit. Med. Journ.* Aug. 1943; Sir W. Langdon-Brown, *ibid.*
Jan. 1945.

they leaned. It left them sadly at the mercy of their own wishful thinking. But to-day the physician employs many facts as clear and sure as those of an engineer. Experiment begins at last to make, as Euripides wished, things talk and tell men what they are.

Fernel's whole life had been densely occupied. His death left MSS. unpublished. Of these Plancy mentions two complete treatises, which he, Plancy, hoped soon to get issued by the press. One was on *lues venerea* and its cure. This disease was the then novel illness, now called syphilis. It had broken out in Europe on the return of Columbus' sailors from the discovery of the New World, 1493. This disease, in the last years of the fifteenth century, was already ravaging all Europe; by 1505 it had spread from Europe even to the Chinese ports. Fernel, in his 'Dialogue' (1548), 'at the request of Brutus'[1] had addressed one of its chapters to the malady. But the later special tractate on the subject, found at Fernel's death, and promised publication by Plancy, had still failed to appear when Plancy died. Although known to a certain circle, it did not reach à printer until 1579. A MS. of it was then secured by the great Plantin press at Antwerp. The work had missed inclusion in the large standard collection of tracts on its subject, published at Venice in 1567 (Collectio Veneta Secunda). The reprint (Venice, 1599) omitted it. So again did the reprint for Boerhaave in Leyden in 1728.

The original issue of this Fernel treatise (1579) mentions that its MS. had reached the Plantin press through Victor Giselinus, a physician and scholar, and travelled man. Giselinus, in a prefatory letter, relates how seven years ago, on his return from Franche Comté (Astruc says he had a doctor's degree from Dôle) to Paris, he found his friend Christopher Plantin had by him a MS. of the unpublished 'De lue venerea' of Fernel. This doubtless was a copy of one of the two treatises described by Plancy as complete at Fernel's death. But, says Giselinus, the MS. had been written by some ignoramus so faultily as to be in places unintelligible. Now, however, that, after eighteen years of travelling, Giselinus has come home at last to his own country (he is writing from Bruges), he has met with an excellent MS. of the work in the possession of Dr Francis Rapard of Bruges. Hence the present volume from Plantin's press.

As for Rapardus he seems to be the Francis Rapaert who[2] had

---

1 Brutus exclaims how glad he would be to hear from Eudoxus about the strange new disease. Bk. ii, c. 14.   2 Astruc, *De Morb. Vener.* ii, p. 198.

published, in Antwerp, in 1551 a counterblast to the then new astrological almanac of Bruges (magnum et perpetuum Almanach, etc.),
for which Peter Haschard of Flanders and Peter van Bruhesen,
physician to Eleanor of Austria, had been largely responsible. The
almanac had urged that astrological auspices not only for bleeding,
purging and bathing should be observed, but that the barbers should
be restricted to astrologically favourable days even for shaving—
including of course the tonsure. The Magistracy of Bruges had
officially endorsed this. Rapaert's tractate asks scoffingly whether
Bruges expects the civilized world to follow her in this lead.

Victor Giselinus, so the omniscient Astruc records, was born at
Sandfort near Ostend in 1543, and studied at Louvain and Paris. He
was a friend of Justus Lipsius. He had travelled in Italy and elsewhere.
He says of Fernel in this preface, 'his works, often printed, are sought
so eagerly that it would seem no one practising medicine can go
without them, and all who would learn its elements must turn to
him'. The tract refers in its text to the year 1556. It would therefore
be written between then and the spring of 1558, when Fernel died.

Fernel dealt with syphilis in three of his writings: the 'Dialogue',[1]
some time prior to 1542; the 'Pathology',[2] 1554, and this tract, 'On
the best cure of lues venerea'.[3] The name 'syphilis' was not current in
Fernel's time. Fracastor's famous poem,[4] christening the disease by
the fanciful name 'syphilis', appeared in 1530, but the name did not
come into common use until the eighteenth century; the pages of
Astruc's monograph make that clear. In Fernel's time the disease
went, professionally and popularly, by many names—Neapolitan
disease, Spanish disease, de las bubas, malum franciae, morbus gallicus,
'the disease from the Indies',[5] mal serpentino, scabies gallica, etc.
Fernel[6] says the french call it the 'neapolitan disease' and the Neapolitans call it the 'french disease'. Morbus gallicus was perhaps the
name most in vogue. But Fernel never employs it, nor does he indeed
any of those others. He designated it, formally and scientifically and

1 Bk. ii, c. 14.   2 Medicina: Pathologia, bk. vi, c. 20.
3 In the Utrecht edition of the collected medical works it is to be found inserted
between books vi and vii of the 'Pathology'.
4 De morbo Gallico sive de Syphilide, Verona.
5 Monardes, Historia Medical de las Cosas, etc., Seville, 1574, p. 14.
6 De Luis Ven. Curat. c. 2. This statement by Fernel repeats the title of Leonicenus'
treatise, De Epidemia quam Itali Morbum Gallicum Galli vero Neapolitanum vocant,
Aldus Manutius, Venice, June, 1497, 4°.

always, *lues venerea*. Perhaps if his treatise *De Luis Venereae Curatione* had not lain unprinted for over twenty years the name *lues venerea* would have been the established one to-day. He was, as we know from a passage in his 'Pathology', careful about the nomenclature of disease, and of diseased conditions. As a writer and teacher of systematic medicine he had to be. His choice of *lues venerea* was significant in several ways.

The sudden outburst of the new disease which alarmed Europe in the final years of the fifteenth century was common talk in all circles, high and low, physicians and laity alike. The theme produced a great crop of printed tracts and treatises. The press became busy almost for the first time with something other than liturgies, patristic texts, sermons, and the classics of humane letters. A cloud of witnesses found in the printing-press a means for airing views and news about the scourge. Gossip of course made free with it and its victims. The printed booklets about it bore dedications to persons prominent in society. De Bethencourt of Rouen was an exception in not dedicating his tract to a specified name, lest doing so beget a scandal. But, for the most part, there was little such precaution because there was little such prejudice. Ulrich v. Hutten inscribed his account of his own case to Albert, Cardinal Archbishop of Mainz; Diaz de Isla dedicated his tract to John III of Portugal; Nicolas Massa his to Carlo Borromeo, Cardinal Archbishop of Milan; and Gaspar Torella his to Bishop Louis de Bourbon. The state of things seems to give additional likelihood to the inference that the disease had it been abroad then would not have escaped mention by Poggio's *Facetiae*. It was said[1] with

---

[1] J. Alex. Brassicanus, Πᾶν, *Omnis*, 1519, Haguenau: Thos. Anselm for Joh. Knobloch, 4°. Brassicanus was a scholar, memorable for studies in greek and a professor at Vienna. The above is a volume of latin elegiacs. One set is addressed to Wendel Fabritius, Professor of Sacred Theology. The author commiserates with the latter on his (Fabritius) having contracted 'morbus gallicus'. He cheers him by saying that he himself (Brassicanus) once had the malady but is cured. It would seem, he says, that poets particularly affect the disease. He mentions contemporaries, Bebelius, Locher, Hutten, 'and many others', in evidence. This was published in the year of Hutten's description of his own sufferings. The chief poem in the book is somewhat in the style of the poem 'Nemo', ascribed to Hutten. Little or no opprobrium seems to have attached to contracting the disease. Gaspar Torella, physician to the household of Alexander VI (Borgia), mentions in his tract (*Tractatus cum consiliis pudendagram seu morbum Gallicum*, etc. November 1497, Rome, 4°, Peter de Latume) dedicated to Cesare Borgia, son of the Pope, that two of the Borgias have died of it, one the Archbishop of Monteregia. He mentions conversing with Cesare on the sufferings from night pains.

callous levity, that it especially affected poets. Even in clerical circles it carried little opprobrium. It was classed sometimes as an 'epidemic'; it was called sometimes the 'pest', sometimes the 'pestilence', or the 'plague'. This heightened the confusion attending it. The true 'plague' itself was of course at that time a frequent and frightful visitant, shutting down whole towns, cities, or even provinces. To mix up with it this fresh disease did not help insight into or measures against either. The orderly mind of Erasmus wondered at there being no established medical name for the disease. We find him, in a letter[1] written in 1525, the year before his death, remarking on 'that disease of uncertain origin, which some call *poscas Gallicæ*, others *poscas Hispanienses*, not yet having found a definite name'. As ever, all that was going on found him alive and quick; but he was not himself a physician. The word he uses in his passing reference to the disease is *lues*.

Among early writers on the disease several were notable scholars. Thus, Nicolas Leonicenus of Ferrara, a friend and teacher of Linacre. His essay[2] does not confuse the disease with *pestilentia*, *plaga*, or *pestis*. Another was Ulrich v. Hutten, a friend of Luther but himself a humanist scholar. He wrote of it not as a physician but as a patient.[3] He had contracted it and was to die of it at the age of thirty-six. Fastidious latinist, he never styles the disease 'pestilentia'. His woeful 'this most pestilential piece of illness', and again this 'pestiferous mischief', are but lay exclamations, not professional description. Jerome Fracastor of Verona,[4] again a humanist, contributed to the theme his famous poem, dedicated to another humanist and poet, Cardinal Pietro Bembo.[5] The poem, even under the licence of verse, does not class the disease either with 'pestilentia' or 'plaga'. Once indeed it does refer to it as 'pestis', but in a way bearing the broad meaning of 'curse'. Apart from 'morbus' used for disease in general, the poem most frequently classes the disease as *lues*. It is when we pass to the north of the Alps that indiscriminating application of 'pestis', 'pestilentia' and 'plaga' becomes usual. Joseph

1 Letter to Christopher à Schydlowetz, Basle.
2 *Liber de Epidemia quam Itali Morbum Gallicum Galli vero, etc.*, Venice, 1497.
3 Hutten, *De Guiaci Medicina et Morbo Gallico*, Moguntiae excusum in aedibus Johan. Schoeffer, 1519, 4°.
4 *De Morbo Gallico sive de Syphilide.*
5 'Asulano', *Rime*, etc.; friend and patron of Augurello.

Grünpeck,[1] Sebastian Brandt,[2] Vochs of Cologne,[3] Widman of Tübingen,[4] Conrad Gilinas,[5] are examples of this and illustrate the confusion. In the 'Elegance in Latin',[6] that favourite glossary by Laurence Valla, whose scholarship detected the 'fraud' of the Donation of Constantine, the two words, *pestis* and *lues*, are specifically dealt with, and their meaning contrasted—perhaps an intentional gloss on the medical writing of the day. Valla says: '*lues* and *pestis* differ, both in genus and species, in this way—when in a town or province fever or some other illness breaks out and seizes individuals, whether men or beasts, such complaint is called *lues*; and so similarly in the case of' trees or crops. But *pestis* kills quickly or passes away quickly from him or what it attacks; and that is called *pestilentia*.' To kill rapidly or pass off rapidly would never be true of syphilis. Valla includes 'beasts', and we have, in Jenner's time, the designation of cow-pox as 'lues bovilla'.[7] The early application of 'pestis', 'pestilentia', 'plaga' to syphilis was a misunderstanding, whether of word or fact or both. Not but that pains were taken by some writers. Thus, Joh. Benedict (*Libellus de morbo gallico*):[8] 'But pest according to Isidore in the *Etymologies*,[9] bk. 4, is contagious and spreads rapidly to many. Whence plainly "morbus Gallicus" is not pestilence.' But Hans Benedict himself soon lapses into styling it 'pestilence'.

Fernel's usage ranges itself, as might be expected, with that of the scholars. His term for the disease is throughout *lues venerea*. He is the to first employ it regularly. An earlier tract had indeed recommended

---

1 Cf. Burkhausen, *Tractatus de Pestilentiali Scorra sive Mala de Frantzos*, s.n., s.l., 1496, 4° (Augsburg, Schaur).

2 Cf. Strasburg, *De Scorra pestilentiali sive Mala de Frantzos*, 1496.

3 *De Pestilentia anni praesentis, etc.*, John Winter, Magdeburg, 1507, 4°.

4 *De Pustulis*; and *De Morbo qui vulgato nomine Mal de Franzos appellatur*, 1497, 4°.

5 *Opusculum de Morbo Gallico*; is in the Luisinus collection, vol. I.

6 *De Linguae Latinae Elegantia*, Rome, 1471, Lignamine. Edition here referred to is second Venetian, 1476, 2°, Jacobeus Rubeus 'of the French Nation'.

7 E.g. Benj. Moseley, *A Treatise on the Lues Bovilla or Cow-pox*, London, 1805.

8 It is in Luisinus, I, p. 140. Astruc dates it 1510.

9 St Isidore of Seville (570–636). Thorndike's *History of Magic and Experimental Science* (I, pp. 623 ff.) remarks that 'writers continued to cite it [the 'Etymologies'] as an authority as late as the thirteenth century'—John Benedict in the sixteenth. Its appeal lay in 'notable power of brief generalization and terse expression'. Dr Klebs (*Incunabula Scientifica et Medica*, p. 180, 1938) lists eight editions before 1501 in the British Museum.

'morbus venereus', in 1527,[1] but its author did not in fact follow his own suggestion, even on the title-page. Not that *lues venerea* is never found in reference to the disease before Fernel. It occurs in the records of the 'University' of Manosque in Provence, as early as 1496. The entry runs that 'the sickness de las Bubas—so the Spaniards call the lues venerea—was introduced here from Dauphiné this year'. This is quoted by Astruc[2] in evidence as to the date of the arrival of the disease in Europe.

The lead given by Fernel in introducing the name *lues venerea* was followed by a number of writers of his own time. The 'Venetian Collection' by Al. Luisinus had in its first issue been called *De Morbo Gallico*; that was 1566, i.e. before Fernel's monograph *De Luis Venereae Curatione* in 1579. But the second issue of the Collection, Venice, 1599, although the same book as before, bore the title altered to *Aphrodisiacus seu de lue venerea*. That Fernel can rightfully be regarded as the reformer in this matter of nomenclature is stressed by Grüner,[3] a medical historian, in 1793. Grüner wrote, 'tandem lues venerea in primis sub auctore Fernelio ut nomen et rei et fonti mali quam maxime conveniret'. The names 'morbus gallicus', 'malum franciae', and their like, must have been distasteful to the French, even as 'morbus neapolitanus' to Neapolitans. Hutten, in employing the former, remarks the injustice of coupling the disease

---

1 *Nova Paenitentialis Quadragesima, necnon Purgatorium in Morbum Gallicum sive Venereum; una cum Dialogo Aquae Argenti et Ligni Guiaci Colluctantium super dicti morbi curationis praelatura, opus fructiferum*, Parisiis, typis Nicolai Savetier, 1527, 8°, by Jacobus de Béthencourt, of Rouen. The book states 'printed from the MS. of the author in 1525'. Rouen suffered, it is said, from an especially severe form of the malady. As to *treatment* of syphilis, this essay is an advance on anything before it. It did not get into the 'Venetian Collection' (1567) or into the Addenda published in 1793 by Grüner. The indefatigable Astruc knew it, and remarks (vol. II, edition of 1760) that the work seemed inaccessible in Germany. Savetier, its publisher, was not prominent, and chiefly dealt with school books. Astruc mentions two copies of the book, one in Bibliotheca Regia—now Nationale—the other in the Sloane Library, London. I fail to trace this latter copy. The British Museum has only the translation into french (Paris, 1871) by the 'syphilogue' Alfred Fourier of last century. In Sweden, Dr Waller has a copy, recently obtained in London. De Béthencourt's *Dialogue* makes Mercury boast: 'I am today admitted to the society of kings, princes, generals, prelates, bishops, and all the great ones of the earth. I cure their ills, even the most incurable.'

2 *De Morb. Vener.* I, bk. i, c. 5, Paris, 1740.

3 *De morbo gallico scriptores medici et historici, partim inediti, partim rari, et notationibus aucti*, collectio edit. DC. Gottfried Grüner, apud Jenam, sumptibus bibliopoli academici, 1793, 8°.

'with the name of a nation than which in our time none is more cultured or more charming'.[1] A similar feeling may have weighed with Fernel. He was substituting for what were merely current nicknames a term logically based on the manner of the contagion. The surgeon, Thierry de Héry,[2] writing in the vernacular as did most surgeons, used 'maladie venérienne' in Paris in 1552, four years after the appearance in print there of Fernel's 'Dialogue'. Juan le Paulmier, Fernel's pupil, employs *lues venerea* in his 'Contagious Diseases'[3] of 1578. Wm Clowes, the Elizabethan surgeon, acquainted with Fernel's treatise on *lues venerea*, writing in England in 1585[4] says, 'in Latine called morbus gallicus or morbus neapolitanus but now properly lues venerea', which seems clearly the influence of Fernel. Indeed, it was one of those twists of fortune which befall words, which let the fanciful soubriquet 'syphilis' oust the logically appropriate 'lues venerea'. True, the less logical was the shorter by three syllables to six; and, perhaps more effective, the very meaninglessness of the fancy term here helping to avoid scandal.

The history of syphilis is a striking example of the problem of how a disease may appear to arise *de novo*. To most instructed, as well as merely popular, opinion in Europe, at the opening of the sixteenth century, syphilis appeared to be a new disease suddenly injected into the world. Some argued, however, that it was really only a vastly increased prevalence of what had long previously existed less noticed because on a smaller scale. Fernel himself inclined to accept the current belief that the disease was *new*, that is new to Europe, and probably brought by the Spaniards from the American islands. He dates it from 1493 'or 1492'.[5] A piece of social evidence signi-

1 *De Guiaci Medicina et Morbo Gallico.*

2 *La Méthode curatoire de la maladie venérienne,* Matthieu David, 8°; and again 1569, Paris, G. Gourbin, 8°.

3 Paris, Den. Duval, 4°. Le Paulmier issued Fernel's Consilia, after Fernel's death. This volume, with its essay on *lues venerea,* preceded by a year Plantin's publication of Fernel's *De Luis Ven. etc.,* which Plancy described as 'finished' at the time of Fernel's death. Le Paulmier seems to have been of Fernel's household along with Plancy.

4 *A brief and necessary treatise touching the cure of the disease called Morbus Gallicus or Lues Venerea by unctions, etc.* 1585, London, printed for Thomas Cadman, 4°. Another edition appeared in 1596.

5 *De Luis Venereae Curatione perfectissima,* c. 11. Bombastus 'the paracelsus', in his tract of 1527, claimed to be the first to write on the disease! Astruc, *op. cit.* p. 126.

ficant that it was new is, I would think, that Poggio's *Facetiae*, dating from 1438,[1] contain, in spite of their theme and character, no allusion to any such complaint. There exists, however, a direct statement by a medical writer in 1500 that the disease had existed, presumably in South Germany, as far back as 1457. The writer was a certain John Widman, physician to the Baths at Wildbad, and he made it in his booklet 'On the Plague and how to escape it'.[2] He is addicted to parentheses, and in one of them he asserts 'the irritating pustules or Asafatis (called malum franciae) which now, from as long ago as 1457 onward to the present year 1500, have spread from district to district with terrible results'. His remark is introduced as if possibly from personal knowledge.[3] He was author of a medical guide to Wildbad Spa in 1513.[4] Astruc gives the year of his death as 1524. He had three daughters already married in 1511. In 1457 he would have been quite young, though perhaps already a student.

A suggestion has been made[5] that '1457' in his book of 1501 is a misprint. There is, however, nothing to support the suggestion. To argue it a misprint because the date is too early for syphilis in Europe is of course to prejudge the very question at issue. There are in London two copies[6] of the book. One of them contains contemporary MS. notes, which do in fact on one page correct a misprint. But the page containing '1457' stands without any correction; the date passed muster therefore under a contemporary hand. The numerals employed for the date are arabic, which are less open to mistake than roman would be. If there were a later edition of the book, that might, of course, supply a test as to misprints in a former edition. A vernacular (german) edition has in fact been said to exist.[7] There is, however, no other edition. The tract in the vernacular (1511), supposed to be a german version of the

1 In print from 1471.

2 Joh. Widman (Mechinger, Salicetus), *De Pestilentia et ejus Fuga*, 1501; Tübingen, 4°; (Joh. Otmar) for F.M. (Frid. Meynberger).

3 He had written on the new disease in 1497 (Strasburg), *De pustulis quae vulgato nomine dicuntur mal Franzos*, a short tract.

4 *Ain nützlichs büchlin von dem Wildpad gelegen im fürstenthumb Wirtenberg*, gemacht von dem berümpten doctor Johann Mechinger, 1513, Tübingen, 4°. The printer must have been Thos. Anselm.

5 Klebs-Sudhoff, *Stud. z. Geschichte d. Medizin*, 1912.

6 British Museum and Royal College of Surgeons.

7 Klebs-Sudhoff, *Die ersten gedrückten Pestschriften*, Munich, 1926, 8°, p. 59.

latin tract of 1501, is in truth a totally different work, though
by the same author, John Widman. Its title is 'What rules to adopt
when plague is in the air'.[1] It is a set of homely precautions against
the plague. Widman's preface inscribes it to his three daughters and
their husbands.[2] The latin tract of 1501 was, on the other hand,
addressed to physicians. The german tract of 1511 is addressed to
lay-readers and is untechnical and popular in style. It was reissued
in 1519. Then again there is in it no reference at all to 'malum franciae'. A supposition by G. Vorberg[3] that the latin tract *De Pestilentia
et ejus Fuga* of 1501 by Widman is itself a second edition is without
support. There was no previous, as no later, edition.

Evidence runs heavily counter to the supposition that the disease
was in Europe before the discovery of the New World. The view,
put forward mainly by Sudhoff,[4] that it was already endemic in
Europe, has not stood critical examination. The contention did not
attach weight enough to the confusion possible where different
diseases, ill-apprehended, were spoken of under merely popular
names. Sudhoff's thesis is contradicted also by pathological material
retrospective over the successive historical periods in question. Human
bones belonging to ancient and medieval Europe, and the mummified
material of Egypt, present no evidence (A. Ruffer) of syphilis. As
to the aneurisms described by the ancient classical writers, they do
not tally with those characteristic of syphilitic disease. On the other
hand, bones from interments in America dating prior to Columbus

1 J. Widman, *Regimen wie man sich in pestilentzischer Lufft halten soll*, 1511, Strasburg, Joh. Knobloch, 20 leaves, 4°.
2 Und umh hit willē derselbē sei/ner döchter menner und Töchter zū gelassen
söl/lichs trücken zü lassen. Damit der gemein unge-/lert man-so nit alweg und zü
vorab in pestilētzi-/schenn Zeiten-gelerter artzer in söllichen zūfellen-/rats zü pflegen
hat-sich zü haltē wyss-in hoffnūg/so die menschen gegen got sich versienen-irlebē
in/götlicherliess anschicken-und der underrichtun-gen in disem büchlin Warnem-
mē-die werden der/sorgfeltigē kranckheit verhütet oder entlediget./Das wol got
barmherziglich mitteylen allen de/nen so dyss büchlin lesen. Der and weg der
reinygung geschicht mit artznye/die die andern böss füchtigkeiten-nit in blüt
vermischt-treibet-es sye galle schleim wasser oder melancoly-davon lass sich ein
yedes vor der Pestilentz purgieren/mit rate eins gelerte erfar-/nē artzet.
Colophon:
Geendet zü Strasburg mitt grossem fleiss/von dem wolgelerten Magistro Mathia
Schüj/rer-im September-nach der geburt/Christi MDxi/
3 Stuttgart, 1924, 4°.
4 *Ursprung von Syphilis*, Internat. Med. Congress, London, 1913. Summing up
his arguments.

bear clear and unmistakable signs of syphilitic disease.[1] Syphilis was
therefore endemic in the New World prior to the visit of Columbus
though not to be found in Europe until Columbus' return thence,

Regimen durch den hochgelerten vnnd übertreff-
senlichen der artznei Doctor Johan wyd-
man/genant Möichinger/gesetzt wie
man sich in pestilentzischem
lufft halten soll.

Fig. 21.

Regimen zů pestilentzischem lufft/georb
net durch doctor Johansen
Meuchinger.

Jeses büchlin haltet inn/eren/wie man
sich halten soll in zerstörtem lufft zů zei-
ten der pestilentz/so uil dẽ gemeinẽ mann
not vnd er begreifflich ist zů vernemẽ/vñ ßwil
die vrsach des sterbens/ist von bösem lufft/faße
ich an am selben/vnd setze dauon etlich Regel.
Die erst Regel/vñ mercklichst/ist das mã sich
byzeit auß dẽ vergifftẽ lufft tůn sol/weyr hinda/
an eẽ ende/da gesond lufft/vñ nyemã da selbs an
der pestilentz ist gestorben/vnd so dan der sterbet
auch dahynn kombt/sol man aber bey zeit fließe
an eyn ander ort/so gesonder lufft/vnd keyn pe
stilentz gewesen ist. Ob aber man dye stethnit für
de/sonder du müßte an ende/da man vor her ge-
storbẽ fliehẽ/so fliße an kein end/da mã kürtzlich
als in dreiẽ monaten oder mynder vngeuerlich
hat gestorben/sonder da man vor lange zeit/als
bey halbem iar/hat vfgeßöret/dan nu ist der lufft
wol daselbs purgiert/von allen gifftrygen dem/
psen/an dem ort behybe so lang biß der lufft an
deinem orte auch wol gereyniget werde/dan kere
wyder in dein hause/oder wonung eigens lufts.
Die ander ist das trüber/dempffiger/mißtiger
vnd füchter lufft/ist diß zeit schedlich/v·nd deß-
halb ist schedlich am mondes schein zů seün.
Die drit regel aller verdempffter lufft/als da
ist/in tieffen wonyngen/ist schedlich.

.21 iiij

Fig. 22.

Figs. 21, 22. Title and text-page of Widman's *Regimen*, 1511.

when it at once broke out in the Mediterranean littoral where he
landed. To clinch the argument further, the record of Ruy Diaz de Isla[2]

1 Williams, *Archives of Pathology*, 1932.
2 *Tractado contra el mal serpentino* (cf. Astruc, *De Morb. Vener.* II, p. 199, edition of
1748, Venice), addressed to John III of Portugal, d. June 1557, and therefore thought
to be *c.* 1555.

has lately come to light, in the National Library of Madrid. De Isla tells how he treated certain of Columbus' seamen for the disease at Barcelona directly on their return from America (Haiti) in 1493. Europe once reached, the contagion spread with speed, and Fernel in 1542 speaks of it as having reached remotest India. Indeed, already by 1505 it was in Canton. 'In the short period of ten years from the siege of Naples this gift from the recently discovered New World circled the Old World completely' (J. J. Abraham).[1] As to the sixteenth-century intensity of the scourge there is the testimony of William Clowes, the queen's surgeon, in his book of 1585:[2] 'It happened in the House of St Bartholomew very seldome, whilst I served there, for the space of nine or ten yeares, but that among every twentie diseased persons that were taken in, tenne of them had the pockes' (p. 2). 'I may speak boldly because I speakee trulie and yet I speake it with very grief of heart, that in the Hospital of St Bartholomew in London there have been cured of this disease by me and 3 others within the space of 5 years to the number of one thousand and more. I speake nothing of St Thomas's Hospital and other houses about the city, wherein an infinite number are dayly in cure' (p. 1, verso).

Fernel was therefore right in judging the disease to be new in Europe and imported from the New World. Very soon after its coming, all classes of society began to suffer from it, from the loiterers in the market place to the College of Cardinals. Fernel remarks[3] that it was worse in Germany than elsewhere by reason of the grosser licence of the way of life there. It seemed to have dropped from the skies. Some thought it an accentuation of disease already known; some confused it with leprosy and elephantiasis, some thought it a pestilence engendered by the stars.[4] Fracastor of Verona taught that it spread by means of air rendered pestilent under adverse conjunctions of the planets.[5] Others traced it to impurity of food. But Fernel said, in effect, 'No: it does not come from the stars, nor from the soil, nor from water, nor from wine. Like the mad dog's phlegm, it is

---

[1] Introduction to H. Wynne-Finch's translation of Fracastor's *Syphilis*, with Notes, London, 1935, 8°. Benivieni (not after 1502) says it is all over Europe, *op. cit. Brit. J. of Surgery*, 1945, p. 225.
[2] *V. supra. A briefe and necessarie Treatise*, etc.
[3] *De Luis Ven. Curat.* c. 4.   [4] *Ibid.* c. 2.
[5] Fracastor, bk. i, 12, 119–25 and ii, 238–48. *V. infra*, Note XIX, *Appendix*, p. 186.

a contagion;[1] that is, it spreads by contact; and it has this further resemblance to the dog's virus that it requires a broken surface in order to establish itself in the body. The sound skin is proof against it; but the least sore place—a scratch, an abrasion, the tiniest crack— and through that it can enter. As with arrow-poison, the sound skin has to be pierced to let it pass. And, like the mad dog's virus, having entered it lies dormant for a while; then, in its own due time, to travel to the uttermost ends of the body, working its mischief as it goes.' This was a shrewd and true observation on a subject at that time in great confusion.

Fernel speaks[2] of guiac as a remedy for the *lues venerea*. Guiac wood was obtained from the New World, and was in great request for the cure. Fernel describes what kinds of specimens of the wood are to be preferred; he finds, contrary to 'Manardus', that the bark is better than the wood. It is unusual for Fernel to advert to a contemporary by name. Johannes Manardus was of Ferrara. He was a commentator on Mesue, and died in 1536.[3] He was author of *Epistolarum Medicinalium*, two of which were on 'Morbus Gallicus', and two more on 'The Indian Wood'.[4] Rabelais edited an early issue[5] of the 'Letters'; they would be congenial to him.[6] One of them says, 'it is better to observe the pulse than the grouping of the stars'. Manardus, like Fernel and Rabelais himself, was 'Aristotelian'. The Utrecht (1656) edition of Fernel, in reprinting the *De Luis Venereae Curatione*, prints the name Manardus as Menardus, both in the text and in the Heurnes' 'marginal' to the text. This might suggest Monardes of Seville, author of 'Remedies from the New World'. But Monardes' work[7] on that subject appeared first in 1565, and Fernel cannot have been writing later than in the spring of 1558. The 1581 edition of Fernel by Wechel prints the name as Manardus.

Fernel, in the *De Luis Venereae Curatione*, mentions another contemporary, the Ferrarese physician, Antonio Musa (1500–55), the name which Francis I, comparing him with the physician to Augustus,

1 *De Luis Ven. Curat.* c. 4.   2 *Ibid.* c. 10.

3 Lecocq's *Bibliotheca.*

4 *De Ligno Indico.* The whole set of these 'Letters' was first published at Basle, 1540, but some had been issued in Paris in 1528, and in Strasburg in 1529; cf. Astruc, *De Morb. Vener.* vol. II, Paris, 1740.

5 Gryphius, Lyons, 1533.   6 *Epist.* ii, 1.

7 *Historia Medicinal de las Cosas se traen de nuestras Indias occidentales,* 1565, Sevilla, Alonso Escrivano, 4°.

gave Brasavola, physician to and friend of Hercules II of Este, and physician to Popes Leo X, Clement VII, Paul III and Jules III. He was physician-extraordinary to Henry VIII of England, Francis I of France and Charles V of Germany. Francis bestowed on him the Order of St Michael, after his publicly sustaining a thesis, *De Quodlibet scibili*, against all-comers for three days in Paris. Brasavola wrote a valued book on simples and other materia medica; an interesting review of it is given by Thorndike.[1] There was a small tractate by Musa—*De Morbi Gallici Curatione*, Venice, 1553. It was on mercury taken internally. It listed two hundred and thirty-four different kinds of the 'Scabies Gallica' as Brasavola commonly called the disease. It was reprinted in Lyons in 1554[2] and again in 1555, and shows Fernel's reading abreast of the time.

Right, as we now know he was, on a number of knotty and at that time debated points concerning this novel and tragic visitation of society, Fernel was yet wrong in one important particular. He judged rightly that the disease was new to Europe, that it came from the recently discovered New World, that it was contagious, not infectious, and could gain entrance to the body only through a wounded, not a sound, surface, that after entry it would lie latent without sign for several weeks, finally to break out, it might be, over the whole system. Where he was wrong was in regard to that most practical of all issues, the cure. He failed to apprehend that a cure was potentially to hand—one of those strange vindications of empiricism which have not been rare in medicine. He did not like empiricism. Moreover, it is surprising that mere empiricism should, in so relatively short a time, hit upon this 'cure' for something altogether novel. Yet so it was. In mercury, simple 'trial and error' had laid its hand on what proved to be a specific remedy for the new disease. Mercurial inunction was being successfully employed against it, by Ant. Benivieni before 1502,[3] by Bartholomeo della Rocca (Cocles) before 1504,[4] and by Berengarius da Carpi perhaps as early. Mercury had already been long in use against obstinate affections of the skin, and skin trouble was one of the most obvious symptoms of the new

1 *History of Magic and Experimental Science*, v, ch. xx, pp. 445–71.
2 *De Morbo Gallico Lepidissimus Tractatus*, Lyons, Sebastian Bartholomew, 16°.
3 *De abditis nonnullis*.
4 *Chryomantie ac physionomie Anastasis cum approbatione magistri Alexandri de Achillinis*, J. Ant. de Benedictis, Bologna, 1504, sm. 2°, transl. into English about 1550.

disease. A formidable complication however accompanied the use of mercury. Introduced into the body, by external inunction or internally by the mouth, it was liable to be 'violently destructive'. In Fernel's phrase it 'dissolved' even the solid parts. 'In those who have had repeated inunctions the strongest bones are attacked, one way or another, by wasting decay. The teeth become loose and black.'¹ And there is purging by profuse salivation, with fetor of the breath, and continuous vomiting and diarrhoea. It is now well known that these malignant effects need not attach to mercury treatment. They can be avoided by using smaller doses, which yet are curative of the disease. That Fernel appreciated this is not clear, either from his special treatise or from his writings elsewhere. He was aware that in contemporary practice mercury was being given so as to do great and even deadly damage. A famous sentence of his *De Curatione* describes how it was administered even to the extent that, on lifting a piece of dead bone, actual droplets of quicksilver were quivering underneath it. John Hunter records a somewhat similar experience.

In his special treatise Fernel described the symptoms proper to the disease and the sequence which they follow. We can compare here his account with other records of that date. There is the autobiographical report by Ulrich v. Hutten.² Perhaps no personal description of a disease contains more poignant tragedy. Hutten, then 31 years old, had contracted it nine years before, and it was to kill him in another five years. Scholar, and friend of scholars (e.g. Erasmus, Melanchthon), religious reformer (friend of Luther), poet, soldier, publicist, travelled courtier, of distinguished presence and good stock, the world had opened to him like a flower. He had found it a sunny place, and was fain of its wonder and beauty. He had felt, to use his own words, 'the joy of being alive'. Then the curse had fallen upon him. He diarized its relentless ravages and his misery. When Fernel practically restates the dolorous picture, it becomes hardly less tragic because in general terms.³

Early in the new century, of treatments competing with the mercurial, one employed the wood of a tree from the New World. A decoction of this was taken internally. It promoted sweating, and was supposed thus to relieve the excess of vicious humour to which, according to the humoral theory, the new disease was due. The wood was known as *ligno santo*, and was from the guiac tree. By some,

1 *Cura de* 1. *ven. c.* 7.   2 The book was placed on the *Index*.
3 It seems gratuitous on the part of Stricker to suggest Fernel as a plagiarist here.

squima, another exotic wood, was preferred; Vesalius esteemed it even above guiac. Fernel for his part taught that the new disease was not truly humoral at all. Its cause, he said, is 'a subtle insensible poison', and the humours merely transport it about the body, but it does not change them. Here, as Le Pileur has stressed, he was putting forward, more clearly than any had yet, an idea which three centuries later became important in pathology.

Fernel, working from his conception of the disease as due to a poison, set about providing an 'antidote' for it. He concocted, with his customary care and skill, a brew of some two dozen selected herbs; he prescribed this 'anti-venereal sedative'[1]—*opiate* he called it, but it contained no opium. For use along with it he made another brew of some twenty other species of herbs, and to this were added certain quantities of the two old-time antidotes 'mithridate' and 'theriac'. On this coupled pair of herbal recipes he relied against the new malady. Nor did he exclude guiac from use, at the same time— it might open the pores of the body and assist the travel of the herbal antidotes to all parts of the system. But Fernel did not resort to mercury. He must have rejected reports widely current about its efficacy. Did the circumstance that the ancient world judged it to be a poison, unduly deter him?[2] His mistake is difficult to excuse. It was a mistake which was to cost his posthumous reputation dear.[3] It was a strange misjudgement, for, in his own words, 'the surgeons are persuaded that mercury is the one sole antidote for the disease'. Among surgeons who were saying so—and saying it in print—were Thierry de Héry,[4] one of the best of the King's 'barber-surgeons',

1 The night-pains of the new disease were said to be 'atrocious'. Fernel quite commonly applies the term 'opiate' to remedies containing no opium. J. Riolan père says 'the soft electuary is commonly called "opiate", not because it contains opium but because it has the consistence of opium'. *Methodus Bene Medendi*, p. 323, Montbéliard, 1588. Theriac was an instance of such an electuary.

2 For example, Ausonius *In Adulteram*:

> Toxica Zelotypo dedit uxor moecha marito:
>   nec satis ad mortem credidit esse datum.
> Miscuit argenti letalia pondera vivi,
>   cogeret ut celerem vis geminata necem.
> Dividat haec si quis, faciunt discreta venenum:
>   antidotum sumet, qui sociata bibet.
>
>   *Epigrammaton*, ix, *circa* 300 A.D.

3 E.g. Gulielmus. Vince, A.B. Oxon. Diss., *De Lue Venerea*, Utrecht, 1699, 4°, p. 12.

4 *La Méthode curatoire de la Maladie Venérienne, Vulgairement appellée Gross Vairolle, & de la diversité de ses symptomes*, Paris, 1552, 8°.

and John de Vigo,[1] chief surgeon to Pope Julius II. Fernel would know too that a number of physicians of good repute were testifying in the same sense as the surgeons—Jacopo da Carpi (Berengarius),[2] Wendelin Hock[3] (1514) and, nearer home, Jacob de Béthencourt[4] of Rouen (1527) where the disease had been notoriously violent. Peter Matthiolus of Siena[5] was even using it internally (1535). It is not to be doubted that at the very time of Fernel's abstention from it more physicians were in favour of the mercurial treatment than were against it.

In support of his own herbal remedy Fernel adduces an observation certainly open to criticism. He says, 'Under their use I saw the destructive ulcers on the patient's face begin to heal in a few days'; and in the next sentence adds that, along with the herbal sedatives used internally, he applied externally to the sores on the patient's face his 'divine water' as a lotion. On turning to the recipe for his 'divine water' we find it contained mercury in the form of sublimate. When Francis I lay dying of the disease, Fernel's opposition to treatment by rubbing with mercury came under public comment. A story went that at a consultation over the king, at which Fernel still urged his specific brew of herbs, Antonio Gallus, one of the Court physicians, interjected, 'He got it in the same way as his subjects, and, as with them, mercury will take it away.' And the remark passed into history.

It was in 1558 that Fernel died, of a fever. He had become physician-in-chief to the king in 1556, on the death of Master Louis de

1 *Practica copiosa in Arte Chirurgia, nuper edita a Johanne de Vigo*, Rome, 1514, 2° (the two opening chapters).

2 *Isagogae breves in Anatomiam humani corporis*, Venice, 1522, 4°. Chap. on tonsils 'in morbo gallio'. Da Carpi was so successful with quicksilver inunctions that he died worth, besides silver, 40,000 scudi. 'All water runs to the sea', adds Fallopio.

3 *Mentagra, sive Tractatus de causis, praeservativis, regimine & cura morbi Gallico, etc.*, Cologne, 1514, 4°; Lyons, 1524.

4 See above, p. 125, footnote 1. This remarkable tractate draws a reasoned comparison between the guiac and the mercury treatments and concludes definitely in favour of the latter. It shows greater insight into the disease than any other of the tracts published up to the end of the first half of the sixteenth century. The author says he has not inscribed it to any patron because it might expose its patron to some social suspicion.

5 Cf. Gaillard, *Histoire de François I*, p. 191.

Bourges. The confidence of the king in Fernel's skill was a by-word at court. In 1557 Henri joined his army for the campaign against the English; Fernel went in attendance on him. The king's quarters shifted continually. Fernel was finishing his 'Cure of Fevers'; he persevered in writing something towards it every day. The winter came, and proved hard. Calais was taken on 8 January, after, remarks Plancy, having been in the hands of the English a hundred years—in fact more than two hundred. Fernel returned to Fontainebleau. There in the early spring his wife fell ill of fever, and died. A little later he himself was taken with fever. It proved fatal. As death approached he showed great concern at leaving his 'System of Medicine' uncompleted, and especially that portion of it dealing with treatment. He made his will on 23 April, J. Barjot and J. le Paulmier being two of the three witnesses of its execution. On 26 April 1558, the eighteenth day of his illness, he died. Friends and colleagues had to the last lavished care upon him. The king and the whole court, says Plancy, mourned for him. He was buried in Paris in the Church of St Jacques-la-Boucherie—now demolished except for the 'Tour' St Jacques.[1] An engraved copper plaque was later put up near the choir; it gave his age as fifty-two; it should have said (Goulin) sixty-one.

Fernel was of the Renaissance. We saw how, as a young M.A. of the University, he practically re-educated himself in order to qualify, so to say, in humanism. His writings, except the very earliest, were in a latin which earned the praise of a humanist scholar of repute.[2] He had the verve of the Renaissance. His preface to the 'Dialogue' is alive with it. 'The world sailed round, the largest of earth's continents discovered, the compass invented, the printing-press sowing knowledge, gun-powder revolutionizing the art of war, ancient MSS. rescued and the restoration of scholarship, all witnessing to the triumph of our New Age.' It was in this spirit that Fernel, when at length he turned toward medicine, felt that an aim for this all-conquering age should be the completion of medicine itself. It was a task to be undertaken on the lines of the great Justinian codification and digest of the Law. A codification of medical knowledge practical and theoretical. In the process of it errors and con-

1 The church was sold for demolition at the time of the *Convention*. The good sense of an architect saved the tower, now the property of the Municipality of Paris.
2 Plancy.

tradictions which had crept in were to be expunged. Not only the erroneous but the equivocal must go. Logic must reign. Galen and all the rest must be radically overhauled and checked against observation. True, the Arabs at best would remain Arab, and were outside humanist scholarship. But these changes once made, there would exist at last, and for the first time, a corpus of medicine perfect and complete.

In that spirit, using the intervals between practice, he sat down to compose his *Medicina*—as in a sense a public duty to the great New Age he lived in. His life, however, was not to be spared to complete his task. At forty-five he published the first instalment, and at fifty-seven he issued a second. Dedicating this latter to the king whose physician he then was, he wrote:

> If I have not succeeded to the extent of my desire, I yet feel I have made some approach. From the approved opinion of antiquity, and after digesting all that has been written contributing anything lasting in philosophy and medicine, I have gathered together, not merely the supposititious and the ingenious, but what is true, solid, and established by good evidence, whether greek, latin, or arab, and added to it further what my own observation has noted to be helpful to the art of healing. All this I have brought together. As to the contentious I have expressed my mind freely. I have not pinned my faith to any single authority, lest I presume too much, or support the mistaken. I have settled disputes; I have resolved doubts; I have removed obscurities; I have laid secrets bare; I have incidentally added new things which had not been understood. For all this at many places I have given reasons, evidence, facts, proofs, assertions, and instances. Nor have I followed speculation alone or experience alone.[1]

King Henry seems to have been aware of this task which Fernel had set himself, and to have taken a sympathetic interest in it. Other contemporaries too followed its progress. Crato of Kraftheim, one of the emperor's physicians, spoke of it as an 'isagogue' or '*the* isagogue'. After Fernel's death, when Plancy had written to Crato complaining of Crato's incorporating Fernel's words in his own writing, Crato wrote back that he had done so because to Fernel's system all physicians resorted as authority. He goes on to relate how Bassiano Landino, on picking up Fernel's *Medicina* in Crato's house, stayed the whole day reading it. It was perhaps one half the length of Avicenna's Canon. On being asked by Crato what he thought of it, he replied 'this Frenchman is greater than Avicenna'. Thomas

1 Letter to the king, prefixed to the *Medicina*, 1554.

Jordan said of Fernel, 'there is no one like him...he is the Hercules of our Augean stable'. Gabriel Fallopio, of Padua, wrote: 'We have the failing, we italians, of belittling the great. But Fernel, if we forgive him his disregard of ancient authority, we must admit to be the greatest physician and philosopher of this age.' In the next century Guy Patin looked back to him as the 'refounder of Medicine'. It was in that light that the Renaissance at his death had come to regard him, and the view persisted long.

The Renaissance has become a term somewhat vaguely applied. We use it here to mean that period of literary and artistic revival under classical models, which, starting in Italy in the fourteenth century, reached, and was still in France in the sixteenth urging, Fernel and his contemporaries. It changed a number of things, but brought no change to the *a priori* doctrine or outlook of medicine. The temperaments, the four humours, the quintessence, the contraries, etc., went undisturbed. The Renaissance, with all its social enlightenment, bowed its head under pestilence and fever with hardly further protest than a prayer. The leper's bell still haunted its.highways. On the stricken field the surgeon would dispense a benison and a merciful stab where to-day's surgeon operates and heals almost without risk or pain. The fluctuating welter of sickness that prevailed in town and country was accepted by the Renaissance as man's predestined and enduring earthly norm. More's *Utopia* hints at no relief from it. The Faculty believed medical practice, as they knew it, to be the ultimate possible of learning and skill. The Renaissance physician was often in letters, taste and manners an enthusiast for the new, but in his craft of healing, he adhered commonly to reactionary convention. Tradition tied him to the past as to a quasi-sacred authority. Even so great and original a Renaissance mind as that of Rabelais—one having moreover first-hand contact with the suffering sick—could, voicing as it did new 'motifs' and reforms in much, yet offer no better counsel to the young physician of the time than this: 'soigneusement reviste les livres des médecins grecs, arabes et latins, sans contemne les thalmudistes et cabalistes, et par fréquentes anathomies acquiere-toi la parfaite cognoissance de l'autre-monde qui est l'homme.'[1] Such an intellect, in the sixteenth century of our era, reverts to that primitive myth. Nothing could remind us better how difficult it was when immersed in it, to escape from

1 Rabelais: edition of the Collection Jannet, Paris, Alphonse Lemerre, 1873-4, II, p. 8.

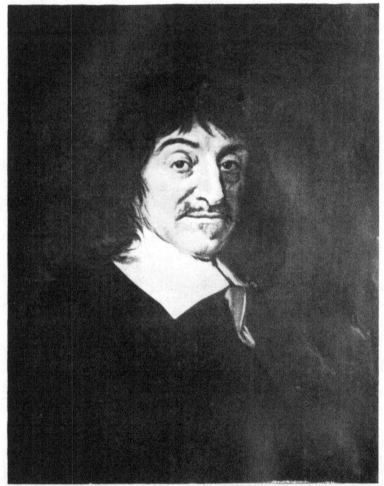

Fig. 23. René Descartes.

that milieu in which Fernel lived, and in which his work was done.

Not until the mid-seventeenth century does a contemporary voice appraise rightly the situation of the medicine of the time and its future—that of Descartes, the philosopher. 'It is true that the Medicine now in use contains little of which the utility is remarkable; but, without having any intention of decrying it, I am sure that there is no one, even among those who make its study a profession, who does not confess that all which men know is almost nothing in comparison with what remains to be known; and that we could be free of an infinitude of maladies both of body and mind, and even also possibly of the infirmities of age, if we had sufficient knowledge of their causes, and of all the remedies with which nature has provided us.'[1]

In Fernel we meet a physician of another and greater order than the scholar-physicians, Ficino, Leonicenus, Champier, Linacre, and others. The idea of a revision of medicine was, with him, of another order than with them.

The greatest of all the disabilities of sixteenth-century medicine would seem not the conflict of opinions between the ancient masters, but the paucity of medicine's assured facts. Crowds of statements parading as 'facts' were uncertainties still to be decided; of solid demonstrable facts medicine had few. The 'renaissance' around Fernel troubled little about this. Intellectually its interest did not lie in probing uncertainties about Nature. Nature had her secrets. That Fernel should be learned in them was the part of a good physician—though that he should eschew help from the stars did seem reactionary and a matter for regret.

Fernel had not the experimental method. Perhaps, it will be urged, he should have turned to it for his purpose. Had the temper of his Age been that of the century which next followed, who knows but that he might have done so. He got his nearest to it, we may think, when, watching illness, he tried to counter it by some carefully adjusted remedy. The spirit of experiment was there. And the problem was there, though this latter in a form so complex as to be hopeless for solution, a bedside-scene crowded with unknowns and variables. Confronting it the physician was the more at a disadvantage because he wrongly supposed he understood it. Only much

1 'Discours de la Méthode', *Philosophical Works of Descartes*, trans. by E. S. Haldane and G. R. Ross, i, p. 120, Camb. Univ. Press.

later did he try splitting it up in order to take factor by factor—that was long after Fernel's century was out.

It may help our estimate of Fernel to place alongside him, for a moment, his after-comer, of three generations later, William Harvey. Three generations is historically no long interval, and these three generations (1554–1616) brought little change to the general position of medicine. For both Fernel and Harvey as students the intellectual setting of medicine was much the same. Neither had any true chemistry to turn to Yet the reactions of the two men to the theory of medicine of the time were quite unlike. This difference, whether inborn or not, is illustrated by the respective reactions of the two to the same story put before them both about the heart. As young men in their respective university schools—Fernel in Paris, Harvey at Cambridge and Padua—they would listen to the same myth about the heart. Both of them would be taught—for it was accepted medical doctrine—that of all distinctions between life and lifeless the most essential is the former's constantly burning vital fire within the heart. It would be expounded doctrinally to them how this 'vital heat', this occult flame, comes originally as a spark transmitted from the stars, an 'innate heat', unlike the heat we know commonly. Not 'elemental' heat, such as pertains to our temperaments and the temperaments of things, but a heat in origin divine, the very principle of life. And that, they would be told, is why the heart is also seat of the imagination.[1] It is the rhythmic upsurging of the 'spirits' of this vital heat within the heart and arteries, which produces the rhythmic life-long pulsation they exhibit, to cease these only at death.

Fernel, instructed in this doctrine, endorsed it. In his maturity, sitting down to write his *Medicina*, he dilated on it. He elaborated more clearly the distinction between the 'vital' heat and the earthly or 'elemental' heat. He straightened out the logical position. He coordinated it more fully with Aristotle. He did for it something like—though he himself would have admitted no likeness—that which Aquinas did in reconciling Aristotle and thirteenth-century Christianity. The 'innate heat and vital spirits' of the classical theory of medicine were, of course, assumptions incapable of demonstrable proof. To-day we should not consider them as resting upon a factual basis. They were, in a word, 'occult'. But, for all that, and for all his

1 *Physiol.* v, c. 77.

critical spirit, Fernel accepted them doctrinally. Sir Thomas Browne, discoursing on 'Life as a pure flame in us', meant no mere metaphor but literal truth. So too I would think for Fernel it stood as literal 'fact'. It had been so accepted for more than 1500 years. Laxity of judgement about 'fact' had been an old failing of medicine down the centuries. Magic was 'fact'. Fernel, it is true, did not accept magic and valued objective fact. Thus, factual exploration of the seats of disease formed the outstanding feature of his 'Pathology'. He cultivated first-hand observation at the bedside, and, less usual still for his time, at the autopsy-table. Sylvius, his colleague, it is said, when an 'anatomy' differed in some detail from the text-book, would complain 'this body seems wrong' and pass on. On the other hand, Fernel—to take the case of the heart—carefully records that, contrary to the teaching of the time, the expansion of the arteries coincides *not* with the expansion of the heart itself but with the moment of its 'contraction'.[1] But he infers from this merely that the pulsations of the heart and arteries are two separate pulsations.[2] He did not follow it further. His was an age when the physician would prescribe in answer to a patient's message, without ever having seen, or intending to see, the patient's self. Fernel himself, according to Plancy,[3] would prescribe at times simply on this plan; but he has in his 'Pathology' sharply condemned the practice.[4] It was a time when—partly owing to the blight of magic—bedside 'fact' went undervalued. Conversely, 'ratiocination' in the study was highly valued; it appraised temperament, predicted 'critical days', estimated the influence of the moon's phase, selected the supposed 'contraries' in medicaments, etc. Fernel endorsed some of this, but he was a living protest against much of it. 'Facts' were welcome to him, just as was talk with men whose direct experience lay in fields outside his own. He said medicine had too few 'facts'.

He welcomed a new fact when it came his way; he made a niche for it in his 'system'. But he did not, as did Harvey, spend hours and days in worrying out a fact in answer to some question it might settle. It was for the sake of 'facts' that Harvey turned to experiment. One thought led to another, and one experiment led to another, and finally one new fact led to another. Teasing his mind about the 'how' of the ways of the body, Harvey, where he could, submitted his

1 *Physiol.* vi, c. 16.
2 *Physiol.* vi, c. 16; *Cordis et arteriorum pulsationes distant.*
3 Plancy's *Vita.*   4 *Pathol.* iii, c. 17.

reflections to factual test. He tried by experiment to get a plain 'yes' or 'no' to the question he had in his head. He laid under contribution 'slugs, snails, scallops, shrimps, crabs, crayfish and many others, nay, even wasps, hornets, and flies'. Thus it was that, 'after observing it in small animals, the frog and the little transparent water-snail, the embryo-chick', etc. he asked himself whether the heart was not just a muscular pump which drove the blood onward along the arteries, and through the veins back to the heart. 'I began to think whether there might not be a movement, as it were, in a circle.'[1] Gradually 'using greater and daily diligence and investigation, making frequent inspection of various animals', he came to the conclusion that he had the truth of it. But he assured his every step by demonstrable fact as he went along. For instance, 'it is shown by the application of a ligature that the passage of the blood is from the arteries into the veins'.[2]

To-day when resort to experiment in medical enquiry is ordinary routine procedure, we may have difficulty in appreciating to the full the originality of mind demanded for such a step in the early seventeenth century. Medicine and biology had drawn little help from experiment for above 1000 years. Only three generations prior to Harvey, Fernel did not look to experiment. It was not that to Harvey was vouchsafed any new technical means, making possible the momentous discovery he made. Harvey had no tools except those which had been to hand from Aristotle's time, and before, onward—scalpel, scissors and thread. It seems perhaps remarkable that Aristotle, or Galen, or some other enquirer, had not already, during the long centuries prior to Harvey, reached the true meaning of the heart and blood-vessels and discovered the 'circulation'. That no one had done so certifies the exceptional nature of the step. After all, what had been lacking through all those previous centuries, not being the means, must have been the man. Essential to a great discoverer, in any field of Nature, would seem an intuitive flair for raising the right question. To ask something which the time is not yet ripe to answer is of small avail. There must be the means for reply and enough collateral knowledge to make the answer worth while. It is significant that the question Harvey put was a mechanical one, not a chemical one. For the latter there was as yet little or no chemistry to tackle it with. Harvey's choice of enquiry suggests that to him

1 *Exercit. Anat.* c. 8.   2 Lecture Notes of 1616, Brit. Museum.

that situation was, so to say, self-evident; though not to Vesalius. He put a straightforward question in mechanics, a study already well advanced. He demonstrated the heart and blood-vessels and blood to be not a fount of 'fire' but hydraulic apparatus. The new-found meaning had significance in many ways, not least in its repercussion upon a young philosopher, Descartes, from whom modern psychology may be said to start.

Hardly less noteworthy than the questions which Harvey asked are some of those which he did not ask—though perforce present to his mind since Fernel, for instance, had dealt with them copiously in his 'Dialogue' and *Medicina*. 'What are the "vital spirits"?' 'Whence are they?' 'What is their relation to the spirits "natural" and "animal"?' 'What is their connection with the "innate heat"?' These questions are nowhere to be found in Harvey's. 'Exercitatio'. Why? He would feel they were not open to demonstrational answer. Asked as to what, during his years of observation of the heart and arteries, he had seen of the 'vital spirits', he replied that he had never met with them. Twenty years later, dealing with Riolan the Younger's 'objections' to the 'circulation', and therefore of necessity entering into doctrinal statement, Harvey abruptly interrupts himself with the remark that to continue further about the 'vital spirits' would be 'tedious'. Such unceremonious dismissal of the 'divine heat of life', within its shrine, the heart, would to Fernel have seemed near to impiety. Further, it would have been a trespass against 'reason', since this argument of the 'innate heat' and its 'vital spirits', had been arrived at studiously by the exercise of logic and 'reason'.

Thus Harvey is widely separate from Fernel. Fernel, it would seem, in order to do his work, must find it part of a logically conceived world. His data must be presented to him in a form which, according to his own *a priori* reasoning, hangs together. In that demand of his lies his inveterate distrust of empiricism. 'We cannot be said to know a thing of which we do not know the cause.'[1] And under 'cause' he included not only the 'how' but the 'why'. With Harvey it was not so. When asked 'why' the blood circulated, his reply had been that he could not say. Fernel welcomed 'facts', but especially as pegs for theory; Harvey, whether they were such pegs or not, if they were perfectly attested. The doctrine of medicine of the sixteenth century used many of what Newton,[2] calling them *hypotheses*,

1 *Physiol.* ii; praef.   2 Cf. Singer, *Short Hist. of Science*, p. 255.

excluded. Fernel got rid of almost all magic and astrology. But there were mysteries, for instance that of the heart, long since explained by traditional appeal to the occult; to many of these Fernel gave his allegiance. And if, as the wise have often insisted, truth is likelier to emerge from reasoned error than from confusion, Fernel, even so, was still a preparer of the way. We may feel he had more love of coherence and order for its own sake than had Harvey.

From two great fields of untidy thinking, however, Fernel came latterly to keep aloof, and did so more and more the longer he lived. One of them was 'natural magic'. It asserted the not infrequent intrusion of the anomalous into the ways of Nature, under praeter-natural compulsion. Fernel, from long and earnest study of Nature, became more and more convinced that, let what may have happened in the past, the present in which he lived offered to the thoughtful mind no departures from an unbroken reign of 'natural law'. Inviolability of natural law was for him one of the great stays of the Universe, and he grew to believe it one of the greatest assets of man-kind.

The second great superstition which in course of time Fernel came to reject utterly was astrology. It saw in the movements of the heavenly bodies a system of extraneous arbiters of human life and fate. Entrenched, no less than magic, in the tradition of antiquity, astrology had, more recently, been fortified by much calculation and science. Renaissance medicine gave way to it almost as an addict to his drug. Fernel, well qualified to judge of its observations from actual experience, had come gradually to recognize that it spelt delusion, and to deal even with plague and epidemic without appeal to the skies. He argued them to be earthly poisons escaping sense.

· Two things were to happen by the middle of the next following, the seventeenth century, after which the old *a priori* medicine would never, and never could be, the same again. The heart, instead of a hearth supporting a vital fire, became a little hydraulic power-plant. And next, at the hands of Descartes, that ghostly tenant, which had long been thought of as the prime mover of the body from within, would be discharged and evicted; the corporeal frame would become simply additional material geared into the movement of the rest of the material universe.

˙ In his pursuit of these and like problems Harvey was an early instance of the new-found delight in natural observation for its own sake, which, somewhat unaccountably, arose as a scientific force in western Europe in the seventeenth century. It had almost the quality of a sentiment—an emotion—and it has endured and prospered ever since. In nineteenth-century Paris Magendie likened his feeling for fact to the zest of a *chiffonier* seeking odds and ends, even from the pavement. A new value began to attach to natural fact. Fernel was a harbinger of this. It shows too in the greater caution with which he accepted 'fact'. The pages of medicine had for centuries been strewn with statements given as 'facts' which were in truth untested assertions. Fernel's writings show a new caution in the endorsement of such dicta. To turn from Fernel's 'Pathology' to, for instance, Benivieni's, the favourite earlier work, is to be struck by this difference. Assertions masquerading as facts are far less frequent in Fernel. On perceiving the scale of this change we also realize the importance of it as a reform. As far as my reading goes, it had been little attempted hitherto. The impulse to undertake it may well have risen spontaneously within Fernel himself. There had often been a noisy discontent with medicine; indeed, it would be true to say, there had always been. Fernel knew it well and knew well that it petered out commonly in temporary resort to superstition yet grosser than before.[1] It commonly attacked some 'view' in medicine in order to replace it by another which it called a 'cure'. But Fernel's reform went behind all that, to the facts behind the 'view'. They were often facts which would not stand careful examination. Fernel was out to exclude all that he did not think testworthy. What he excluded belonged—we see when we look back—mainly to two distinct though related classes, the magical and the astrological. He had reached the conclusion that magic and astrology, imposing though they might be, were for their most part simply collections of loose thinking. Fernel gradually judged them to rest upon false 'facts'— the direst element of confusion in all medicine. He therefore excluded magic and astrology almost completely from his medicine. That was no easy line to take. It bade defiance to two ancient systems of learning which had intermeddled with medicine even from the

1 E.g. the 'Paracelsus'. L. Thorndike, resuming the work of 'Paracelsus', says with justice: 'In short for Paracelsus there is no such thing as natural law and consequently no such thing as natural science. Even the force of the stars may be side-tracked, thwarted or qualified by the interference of a demon. Even the most hopeless disease may yield to a timely incantation or magic rite.' *History of Medicine and Experimental Science*, v, p. 628, 1942.

oldest times. Their authoritative omission from medicine by Fernel was an advance toward the enlightenment around us now. He has his place among those to whom is owing such freedom of rationalization as we enjoy to-day.

And so we take our leave of Jean Fernel. His days were taxed, year in year out, to meet an overwhelming professional practice, and he gave himself to its cares and its exacting routine in no unwilling spirit. But, through all, he was one who never let himself forget that the sick man lay against the great background of living things in general, and the stars and a Deity beyond the stars. He was also one who, amid an age of furious currents of opinion, never relaxed his effort to read Nature without fear or favour, and judge what may be the rightful grounds of the dignity of man. It seems worth while, across the centuries, to seek contact with such a one, and, as we do so, the temptation is perhaps to pick out, in the light of to-day's knowledge, what has proved right in his outlook, and to exalt it, that its worth may shine the brighter. But there, I think, he would have been the first to smile and say, 'if you value me, do me the favour to render me all in all for what I was. I was right earlier than my time in some things; I was compact of mistakes too. If I live, let me live in the round and altogether.'

Appendix

NOTE I. BIOGRAPHICAL NOTICES OF FERNEL.
GUILLAUME PLANCY (p. 2)

OF biographical notices of Fernel the most important is the 'Life', in latin, by his younger contemporary and follower, Guillaume Plancy. It was written almost certainly some fifteen to twenty years earlier than the short account given by André Thevet in the *Vrais Portraits*, 1583; but it was not printed until 1607. Brief though it is, it yet forms the chief source of the biographical accounts since its issue. Pierre Bayle[1] seems, however, in error in supposing it was the source for the notice by Thevet, unless Plancy's *Vita* had, in some way, become accessible in MS. to Thevet. The issue of the *Vita* which Bayle himself used contained the marginal 'reginam curavit'; it therefore was not one of the early issues. Bayle rightly comments upon that marginal as incorrect; he attributes it to 'the publishers'. The Leyden edition (1646) and the Utrecht (1656) contain it, and it is thought to have been supplied by the Leyden physician, Heurnius, who annotated those editions. Bayle speaks of the *Vita* as to be found in all the editions of Fernel's collected works; but some of the Geneva editions do not contain it, nor do any editions before 1607. Goulin, in his *Mémoires Littéraires* (Paris, 1775), annotated the *Vita* liberally, and translated it into french.

As to Guillaume Plancy himself, his date of birth is given as 1514. He described himself 'Cenomanus', i.e. of Le Mans. He was, according to Goulin, taking his Licentiate course for Medicine in Paris in 1552-3, and proceeded to his M.D. in 1554. He himself states that he lived in the house of Fernel for ten full years. He seems to have been present[2] at the final scene at Fontainebleau, 1558, so that he would have joined Fernel's household about 1548. A remark he makes on what Fernel was engaged in writing in that year agrees with the supposition. Goulin finds Plancy's name in a list of the Medical Faculty of Paris for 1565; he issued his edition of Fernel in 1567. He had translated Synesius and Chrysostom, Paris, 1547. In 1551 he issued the greek text of *Galen's Commentary on Hippocrates' Aphorisms*, Lyons, 8°, and in the same year *Plutarch's Feast of the Seven Wise Men* (greek and latin), Andreas Wechel, Paris, 4°. Wechel was at that time Fernel's printer and publisher. Of Plancy's *Galen on Hippocrates* there were at least five reissues (Paris, 1555, 8°; Lyons,

---

1 *Dictionnaire Historique et Critique*, vol. II, 1136, Amsterdam, 1697.
2 He uses the 1st person when describing the autopsy, in the 'Life'.

1561, 8°; Paris, 1582; Geneva, 1595; Paris, 1637). He wrote the greek couplet which was printed under Fernel's portrait in the editions of the *Medicina*, 1554, etc. He had been a pupil of the Renaissance scholar, Guillaume Budé. He was entrusted with the editing of Budé's 'Letters in Greek', a collection published (by Wechel) in the year of Budé's death, 1540. He was literary executor also to Fernel. (Cf. J. Lamy, in letter from Paris, September 1577, in the introduction to the *Method. Gener. Curar. Febrium*, in the *Universa Medicina* (of Wechel 1567).) In 1567, nine years after Fernel's death, Fernel's *Medicina* was reissued by Wechel as the *Universa Medicina*, edited by Plancy. Plancy is not traceable after 1568. He was no longer alive in 1574, when Andreas Wechel, formerly of Paris, reprinted the *Universa Medicina* at Frankfort, whither Wechel had removed, in 1573, on account of religion. John Crato's letter in that edition refers to Plancy as being dead. Goulin had heard that Plancy died in 1568.[1]

Plancy lived under Fernel's roof when the latter was writing his *Medicina*. He was entrusted, he tells us, with searching the ancient authorities for their accounts of drugs. Fernel would then check that information against his own experience, and finally state his considered therapeutic view in the *Medicina*. Plancy, in the Preface to the 'Universal Medicine', evidently had two things much at heart. One, the bitter and bloody civil strife between the opposed religious parties, into which his country was divided. It was the year before the 'Revolt of the Netherlands', and still five years to 'St Bartholomew's'. His other distress was the ill-feeling and injustice still prevailing in the Faculty of Paris in the matter of Fernel and his teaching.

As to the biographical notice of Fernel by André Thevet (Paris, 1584), it is only five folio pages long, but it supplies a useful control for the short 'Life' by Plancy, the other contemporary account. Not that I know of any reason for doubting Plancy's general accuracy, but there is evidence for supposing that his MS., published so long posthumously, was not in good condition when ultimately printed at Frankfort. Thevet's account agrees closely enough with Plancy's 'Life' to prompt us to ask, as Bayle did, whether the latter, certainly the earlier written, had not been seen by Thevet. That seems unlikely, for presumably its MS. left Paris for Frankfort in 1573, when the Wechel firm removed thither. There may of course have been more than one MS. of it. No mention is found in Thevet of the jealous hostility of the Paris Faculty toward Fernel, borne witness to by Lamy and Capell as well as by Plancy himself. Thevet, as outside the medical profession, may not have been aware of it, although Plancy, Lamy and Capell as physicians were so. Thevet is reputed an unreliable writer.[2]

1 Hirsch's *Biogr. Lexikon* gives 1610!
2 L. Seinèan, *Problèmes littéraires du Seizième Siècle*, Paris, 1927, p. 149.

Shorter biographical notices of Fernel are to be found in Sambucus,[1] Paschalus Gallus[2] (Pascal Lecocq, of Poitou), de Thou,[3] A. Chalmers,[4] P. G. Boisseau,[5] C. S. Saucerotte[6] and by Le Pileur in his preface to the text and translation of the *De Luis Venereae Curatione Perfectissima*, Paris, 1879. There is also L. Figard's *Un Médicin Philosophe au XVIe Siècle* (see chap. 1), Paris, 1903; and A. Rittmann. This last is prefixed to a summary (*Culturgeschichtliche Abhandlungen über die Reformation d. Heilkunst*, III, p. 88, 1869-70: Brunn) of Fernel's purely medical writings. It is drawn briefly from Plancy's 'Life'. Rittmann compares usefully Fracastor with Fernel. He says the edition of Fernel available to him is the Utrecht, 1656, which he calls the 14th and last issue of the *Universa Medicina*—but there are extant 32 successive editions and the last is Geneva folio of 1680. Rittmann is unaware of Goulin (1775) on Fernel. He takes the arrangement of the Utrecht edition to be that of the original and seems to suppose the 72 consilia intended as an appendix to the 6th book of the 'Pathology' and the *Lues Venerea*. He misquotes the date of the year given by Fernel as that of the outbreak of syphilis, thus missing Fernel's inference as to it and the discovery of America. He uses without question the marginals supplied in the seventeenth century (by the Heurnes) as though they belonged to the original—e.g. that Fernel is following J. Sylvius in anatomical description.

Plancy's *Vita Fernelii* was first printed in the sixth edition of the *Universa Medicina*, 1607, a 3-volume 8° issue. The 'Life' is in vol. 1. The printers and publishers were Marney and Aubrey of Frankfort and Hanau, successors to André Wechel, formerly of Paris. The 'Life' was therefore first printed when Fernel had been dead forty-nine years and Plancy at least thirty-three years. The MS. used was not in Plancy's autograph. In view of Plancy's known literary accomplishment the 'Life' seems too ill arranged to be as Plancy intended. In one point it seems incorrect[7] and contradictory. Perhaps a part is missing. In the troubled times which fell on Plancy it, likely enough, was not fully revised. The marginal inserted in the original issue, namely, *forse scripsit Lii*—'perhaps he wrote 52'—suggests the MS. was partly illegible. The original must have been written between 1558 (Fernel's death) and 1574, when we know Plancy too had died. The 'Life' is not included in some Geneva editions of the *Universa Medicina*, but is in

1 *Icones Veterum aliquot, ac recentium medicorum philosophorum*, Antwerp, 1574, 2°.

2 *Bibliotheca Medica, sive catalogus illorum qui ex professo Artem Medicam in hunc usque annum scriptis illustrarunt*, 12°, Basle, 1590 (gives Fernel's age as forty-nine).

3 *Historiarum sui temporis*, see lib. XXI, Paris, 1604; Geneva, 1620; edit. E. Buckley, London, 1733.

4 *General Biogr. Dict.* vol. XIII, London, 1814.

5 Jourdain's *Biographie Médicale*, vol. IV, Paris, 1821.

6 *Nouvelle Biographie Générale*, vol. XVII, Paris, 1856.

7 Cf. below, p. 154, 'Life'.

the Leyden and Utrecht editions. The Geneva edition of 1680 is its last appearance. The rendering which follows here (Note II) is from the latin of the Leyden edition (1656), to which a number of marginals were added by the editors, the Heurnes of Leyden. These marginals have been included, though not in Plancy.

NOTE II. PLANCY'S 'LIFE' OF FERNEL
(first printed in 1607) (p. 2)

Birthplace.
Born A.D.
1485

JEAN FERNEL was born at Clermont, a town just twenty leagues from Paris; there he got a good education. He called himself 'of Amiens', however, because his father was from Amiens originally.

Studies classics and philosophy

At Clermont as a grown lad, when he had learned grammar from the schoolmaster, his mother declared it time he turned to business and to the cares of the household instead of to learning. But moved by a passion for letters he begged his father to let him go to study·rhetoric and philosophy in Paris. He promised hard work should make up for lost time. And his father willingly acceded. The old man, with his breadth of experience, knew that, just as in the cornfield good and productive soil promises a fine crop, so likewise with man and learning, passion for study and the budding of innate inclination from youth up presage a maturity rich in bright accomplishment.

At that time there were at the Collège de Ste Barbe in Paris, along with the teachers of the liberal arts, a numerous group of young men not badly (for those times) equipped in learning. Their knowledge and earnestness were a spur, to urge him on all the quicker, to acquire the learning then held in esteem. So much so that the progress he made in the art of disputation in the two years was far greater than he had himself expected.

Noticing he had gone astray in them

Directly he had taken his Master's degree by public examination, the heads of some of the Colleges vied in inviting him, at exceptional salary, to teach dialectic. He declined. He desired to make himself better acquainted with the writings of Cicero, Aristotle and Plato, by private study. It was when he proceeded to do so that he first became aware how far the course and manner of his study had strayed from the true path. All he had done was to pick up futilities inculcated by barbaric tutors. It was, however, a situation which he endured the more calmly, because it was a misfortune which befell the majority, and he recognized it as no fault of his own but as attaching to the age he lived in. Indeed at that time the University of Paris, which we read had been the foremost of all schools which ever flourished since the foundation of the world, was still, as to the Arts, 'barbarian'. Its

grammarians and rhetoricians had in their hands only rude Alexanders, Theopagituses, *Graecismuses*, Theodoletuses and a ruck
of writings of that stamp. Its dialecticians taught from nothing
but the *Termini* of Clichtoveus,[1] the *Summulae* of Peter of Spain,[1]
the *Logica* of Bricotius, and other similar works.

Fernel having suffered this setback at the very start and
threshold (of his study), made up his mind that the path lost must
be regained by diligence and hard work. He resolved to forgo
entertainment, convivialities, feasts and drinking bouts, and even
talks with fellow-students and acquaintance. He took account
neither of food nor sleep nor exercise nor ailments nor affairs; he
put up with everything in order to attain knowledge of the
liberal arts. He dedicated to them all his effort, diligence, care
and industry. He had no other delight than learning. He thought
every hour lost which was not spent in reading and studying
good authors. Desire for learning filled his mind; he was in love
with scholarship and knowledge. *he repaired it by fresh study*

His first care was to free his latin from barbarism—a vice
of the age, which he had caught from ill-read teachers. He
turned especially to Cicero—most of all to his classical speeches
and his discussions on philosophy—and chose the *De Natura
Deorum* and the *De Officiis*. He devoted several months of reading
to obtaining proficiency in narration. Celsus too he admired
very much for his purity of style and solidity of judgement; and
Plato also, whose works Marsilio Ficino had translated into latin. *in classics*

But he was unskilled in mathematics, so that he would stumble
over examples commonly given by authorities in their exposition (of the subject); he felt it a scandal to be ignorant in a field
of learning, which he admired not less than any other. So it was
that he set out to cultivate his mind systematically, apportioning
distinct and separate periods to his several studies. He gave the
morning to arithmetic and mathematics; after the midday meal
he turned to natural philosophy, and after supper to the latin
classics, paying special attention to their style. *in philosophy*

During this insatiable pursuit of letters, toiling unrestingly, he
was at length attacked by a quartan fever. He suffered long and
cruelly. He had to break off his studies, seek healthier air, and
go away.

The quartan fever at length left him. His strength had been
recruited in the country, and he could think of returning to
Paris. He began to talk over with his friends the career he should
take up. Some proposed divinity, some mathematics, some this *At length devoted himself to medicine*

1 This statement is made also in the Notice by A. Thevet (1584).

or that other study to which to give his life. Several urged juris-prudence with its promise of easy circumstances, honours and rank. He was, they said, bound to do well in it, excelling as he did in knowledge of the liberal arts. But, prudent as well as clever, he felt that, in regard to each of all these callings, account had to be taken, in judging the future, of his own individuality, so that, as they say, Minerva be neither rashly nor unwillingly approached. Since he loved solitude and retreat, and was not very apt in expressing himself, he judged he would not be really suited either for the bustle of the courts, or for the assemblies of Holy Church. Therefore it was he chose Medicine in preference to those other fields of learning and profession; also remembering his own recent experience of the boon it could be.

A protest from his parents

But, beside that, while he was thinking over these things, he got a letter from home protesting that the study of one son had already cost over much, and that the others must be looked after no less than he. He must choose between coming home or seeking elsewhere the means of an honest and respectable livelihood. Nor was he at all alarmed at this. He kept on as he was. He thought perhaps to pull through somehow, or perhaps that his father would relent.

Lectured on philosophy

First, therefore, he turned to giving instruction in philosophy, and, this time, not in private lessons within the walls of his own room, but by public lectures in the College of Ste Barbe,[1] and no exercise more sharpens the wits and strengthens the memory. The philosophy course to be covered was that of an age still rude; he got through with distinction and won praise all round. Mean-time he was becoming more and more attracted to mathematics, and the degree to which he carried them is evidenced by the works in them which he published at the time. His written style was, it is true, less fine and polished in them than in his medical writings, but that was the fault of their day. At that time truly, as I remarked before, the language in all our Schools was un-scholarly, and barbaric. The brilliance of a more polished learning had not yet illumined the philosophers of France.

Then completed his medical curriculum

When he had devoted to these studies introductory to medicine more labour than enough, he turned wholeheartedly and with all his might to complete the four-year curriculum leading direct to medicine. Thus, frankly devoted to it, he, both by disputation and by public lecture, gave proof of his outstanding learning.

1 Mentioned also in the Notice by Thevet (1584), who says the lectures expounded Aristotle directly instead of merely through the medium of Clichtoveus and Peter of Spain, and that they made Aristotle clear to every student's understanding.

The first two years of basic work for the doctorate accomplished, when many of the graduands run round soliciting 'a first class' the assembled Faculty and its bigwigs awarded him a second. A 'first' would assuredly have been granted had the furnishing of his purse been equal to that of his head.

The doctorate gained, he settled in Paris, attracted to it by the large number of exceptional men to be met there, their learning and example furnishing instruction and incentive to himself. *Chose to settle in Paris*

For he did not as many, or indeed as most, of us do, so soon as our academical laurels are won, indulge that shallow notion and view of our attainments, which thinks work is now over and that we can take a holiday. No, he did not relax. He turned ever more and more to the classic writers, and the examination of their opinions. About one thing he grew convinced—and he was right; namely, that the knowledge gained from scholastic disputation is only raw, and forms merely a beginning, useless unless developed by further study. He therefore withdrew from all disputation in the Schools, both philosophical and medical, to continue his reading of the great masters for himself at home, and he did that for several years.

In Paris at that time there was a rhetorician of distinction, Jacques Destrebey,[1] versed in the best literature. He approached Jean Fernel, whom he knew to be skilled in mathematics, with the idea of their co-operating. The two exchanged the learning of their respective fields, turn and turn about. Destrebey learned mathematics from Fernel, Fernel the fine flower of letters from Destrebey; and Fernel's style gained in expression, both in dignity and fullness. *Where he cultivated classics*

Meantime he designed some mathematical instruments,[2] and had them constructed, at much cost to himself, and—for he had recently married—dipping into his wife's marriage-portion. Contemplation of the stars and heavenly bodies excites such wonder and charm in the human mind that, once fascinated by it, we are caught in the toils of an enduring and delighted slavery, which holds us in bondage and serfdom. *and mathematics more fully*

His father-in-law, a prudent and accomplished man, often saw his son-in-law, and from time to time had him as a guest. Talk would then turn, between the dishes, to medicine and its problems; he would take occasion to complain to his son-in-law that medicine, which had been his whole devotion formerly, *from which his father-in-law*

1 Also mentioned in this connection in Thevet's Notice of 1584, i.e. prior to the publication of Plancy's 'Life', 1607.
2 Thevet mentions astrolabes among them.

now concerned him too little. He so clung to mathematics that neither love of his wife, nor the endearments of his children,[1] nor the care of his house, could take him off them. 'Now, knowledge of mathematics is in itself as culture well enough, and exercises the wits, if one uses moderation in the time given to it. But it becomes a scandal when an honest man with duties to the public and his family reposes, so to say, to sleep on the quicksands of the sirens, letting the years go by. Mathematics made no contribution to the public weal. Apart from a modicum of arithmetic and geometry it touched society little or not at all. On the other hand when we turn our gaze and thought to medicine we find it a science occupied either with sublime enquiry into Nature or with deeds of beneficence and utility. It is of right the worthiest of all the arts. Mathematics offers no comparison with it.'

and his wife   Senator of Paris and man of experience as he was, he urged on
dissuaded   Fernel these and other good reasons. But Fernel seemed im-
him   movable. The father-in-law, moved by his daughter's tears, lost
his temper and scolded his son-in-law. But we need not enter into that here. Fernel gave way at last, under these entreaties and reproaches. He renounced his mathematics[2] and began to devote himself to medicine with a greater zeal than ever before. Thus it came about that he dismissed the craftsmen and engravers whom he maintained—not without considerable cost—under his roof. He notified some distinguished pupils who were studying mathematics with him that they must look elsewhere for a master, and he disposed of his collection of the writings of all the old mathematicians, and of the astrolabes and many other costly bronze instruments he had devised for himself. He gave himself entirely to medicine.

Returned to   He found that after he had spent a good part of the day in his
medicine he   study, reading and digesting the masters of medicine, he still had
commented   time left over. Lest he should waste it during this period of pre-
Hippocrates   paring himself for practice, he turned his thoughts to expound-
and Galen   ing the writings of Hippocrates and Galen in the public schools, as he had made a beginning of doing even before taking his doctorate. The students flocked to him, and the attendance to

1 Fernel is known to have had two children, daughters, and the younger of them is shown by Goulin not to have been of marriageable age at the time of her father's death, in 1558. But this incident of the relinquishing of mathematics dates in 1535 or 1536. Perhaps Fernel had other children who died young.

2 This story of the abrupt relinquishing of mathematics is similarly reported by Thevet (1584).

hear him was such that in a few years the fame of his learning
went far afield, beyond France to Italy, Spain, Germany, and
throughout Europe. His reputation spread far beyond those who
heard him in the Schools.

When he had spent six whole years in this work of teaching
and practice, and with great success, the fame of his name in Paris
had so grown that he could hardly find time for seeing all the
patients who came to him. They were not Parisians only;
there came strangers who had any serious complaint. This com-
pelled him to give up the teaching he had been doing.

But, that he should not neglect the theoretical part of medicine,
he gave any spare time, which affairs, practice, or business matters
left him, entirely to composing a treatise on the part of medicine
which he styled 'Physiology', illustrating it by comments and
reflections. In this remarkable treatise he surpassed himself.
Generations to come, freer from envy than this of ours, will
perhaps do it justice more openly. He was the first, so far as I
know, to drive out of the Schools those futile mystifications, the
stigmata of an uncultured age, in the form of questionaries,
blatant, nasty and couched in barbarian language, inextricable
labyrinths of quibbling and sophistry, whereby things, clear
enough in themselves, become wrapt in blinding obscurity.
This natural part of medicine he expounded fully, and none the
less tersely, in latin. Anyone grounded in the method and principles of philosophy, who wants a separate treatise of that part
of medicine, and will read it through attentively once, and then
once more, impressing it on his memory by reflection, will find
that nothing noteworthy escapes of all that the ancients—greek,
roman, and arab—have in countless volumes set forth, and that
one man in a lifetime could hardly read through once.

On the issue of this book from the press, he was begged to give
lectures on it, by all the young graduands, with entreaties and
gifts. He undertook the task out of good will and the desire to
do his utmost, and especially as a teacher, although his wife, his
friends, and his patients protested, and although he had great
expenses at home. For three years he devoted strenuous work
to this, proving himself an eminently useful citizen of the republic
of letters. From his School there went forth skilled physicians
more numerous than soldiers from the Trojan horse, and spread
over all regions and quarters of Europe.

Meanwhile besides discharging his duties vigorously and con-
scientiously as lecturer, he spent his evenings in writing another
tractate 'On the principles of blood-letting', a work essential
to the physician. It was like his foregoing treatise terse and

[marginal notes:] whence he acquired renown

and medical practice

Cultivated physiology however regularly, and taught it

and commented it

Then wrote on blood-letting

complete; after its issue he at once took it for the subject of his lectures.

Treated the queen[1] He had not finished giving his courses upon it when he was called to the court by a quasi-regal summons to the case of a lady of the highest quality who was very dangerously ill. Report of his great ability had reached the Prince of the Realm, and the repute that, in all France, there was, so to say, but one physician who could contend effectively against her disastrous illness. He was judged to be a puissant protector against the menace of death, and an averter of ills such as was Hercules Alexicacus. And well did he justify that reputation. The lady's life was saved, contrary to all expectation, and although already despaired of she was rescued from the very mouth of the pit.

Summoned to be physician-in-chief The lady was very dear to the prince and this was a main reason why Fernel was always afterwards especially valued by Henry, prospective king of France. The prince at once chose him his physician-in-chief, offering him an annual stipend to remain at court in his retinue, and take over the charge of his health.

Excused himself from that office But with Fernel desire to learn was always stronger than lust after notoriety. He declined the emolument and honour offered by even so great a prince. He could not be persuaded to stay on at court; promises could not win him over, nor was he moved by remonstrances, nor by entreaties, whether of nobles or of friends then frequenting the court. So it came about that he simulated ill-health. He said, further, that he was not yet sufficiently experienced and versed in the art of medicine to fit him to be entrusted with responsibility for the prince's state of health. On that ground he begged the future king's majesty, in all charity, to let him return to Paris where he had to complete the studies he was engaged on, and to accumulate longer and wider experience in the practice of his art. Later he would justify his industry, both to the king and the court.

that he might gain more experience He was fully aware, indeed he often declared, that, in medicine, experience in treatment counts for more than the precepts of the masters. The physician, the military leader, the orator, the lawyer, or indeed the expert in any calling, however well versed in the principles of his art, can accomplish nothing really great, save by practice and experience. He felt that nowhere could he get the one and the other better than in Paris, with the many men of learning gathered there, and the variety of disease incident there.

1 This marginal (? by Heurne) is in error—the patient was Diane de Poitiers.

Further, he judged unworthy of the title of physician those in a great city . who, acquainted simply with the principles and institutes of medicine, set up in practice in some small town, before having obtained long and full experience in some busy and populous city, picking up there a number of things which are urgently desirable he should know, for the due treatment of disease— things which, just as they came handed down to our forefathers from their forefathers, have in that way too to be transmitted by us to those who come after us. For when at times they make a mistake, as is likely enough, about the cause of the disease which among famous physicians is to be traced, or in prescribing for its treatment, who is there to prevent or correct them? It is undeniable—and why not frankly admit it—that to those who have practised long and with deserved success, there accrues a something in virtue of which they excel, a something eminently desirable, but not easily to be obtained from books, nor properly describable in words—to be gained only by observation and lengthy experience.

Accordingly he judged the surest and quickest way of learning Fernel's view of how medicine is to be learned medicine was this. After a thorough grounding in the principles and elements of philosophy, to learn straightway from some terse and well-written medical précis such details as have to be known of the nature of the human body; then to master the flavours, powers and virtues of medicaments simple and compound; and then to learn to distinguish the signs and symptoms of the several diseases and their causes, and to gather these together, as a store within the memory; then, finally, to follow, long and attentively, the art of practice of some elderly practitioner, capable and ex- perienced in treatment, and to observe in the sick patients them- selves what you have read in the books and heard in the lecture- room. He held that there was much in the theoretical part of medicine which could not be explained truly, nor understood, except by way of long practice and experience. He judged that no one can get through on books alone, numerous although books are. The best instructors in medicine were in his view practice and experience; they clear up the obscure and equivocal which so embarrass and obstruct the beginner, and they fortify him. So it was that he dissented from growing grey in following theory, as in fact most do. Rather should one go forward early into the art of practice, since it is of all teachers the best, but in so doing take for guide an old physician of experience.

This way of thinking was a departure from, and indeed the Subtleties especially to be avoided opposite to, the orthodoxy of practically all professors of medicine until his time; so too it is contrary to the error of the present day in which the Schools inculcate, and stress to their audiences, almost nothing but the meanings of technical terms and empty paradoxical word-spinnings.

Excessive ornateness of style

Also he set his face against those who indulge in an ornate style of speech, and out-of-the-way expressions, aiming less at precision than at a flow of sentences. Such exposition studies ornament rather than meaning, and may almost neglect observing and taking note of the things themselves. 'For just as with a piece of money we look to the weight and material rather than to the artistry of its engraving, so with a lecture it is less the nicety of the phrases than the directness and lucidity which convey its meaning.' Hence it came about that of those who had attained elegance and ease of language, philosophers though they were and well versed in medical learning, few had approached the medicine which wanted doing, for the reason that they had given more thought to the ways and embellishment of speech than to the business of curing the sick truly, safely and suitably.

Too much anatomy and botany

Often too I have heard him declare the absurdity of going on toiling, even into old age, in turning over books of anatomy and reading the properties of simples, without ever looking at a sick man or actually seeing the things which the ancients have described in the sick. He argued it is better after perusing once and then once again some skilled and well-written but brief compendium of anatomy, and going through it attentively, to pass straight to the things themselves as they can be seen and observed in numbers of sick persons, and not to lose time, and the years life has to offer, in reconciling a multitude of authors whose statements disagree. To-day, he said, books on anatomy are almost more numerous than are the sick, and there are more writers of herbals than there are herbs to describe.

Languages

He agreed, however, that skill in languages was a means to true knowledge, and was, if used rightly, of very great help to the would-be physician. That is, if it did not make him too proud to learn of an apothecary how medicaments are to be combined and mixed, or of the old practitioner how to treat a patient. But let him not betake himself straight from his books to actual practice, arrogating to himself in his conceit a complete knowledge of medicine. If he do, how mistaken he finds himself, and how mischievous it may be to the patient, and, more, how harmful to the public weal.

The study of forecasting by astrology

Also he considered that the part of astronomy which treats of the motions and revolution of the heavens and the risings, courses and settings of the stars, is always of good use to the physician, and he dealt with it in his published works.[1] But he condemned

1 This is Plancy's only reference to the three first treatises by Fernel.

wholly astrology with its genitures and divinings invented out
of the stars by superstitious observation of I know not what
portents and falsehoods, and erecting certain 'celestial houses and
habitations' for no other reason than to foretell favourable or
adverse fortune from horoscopes, and imagine certain characters
and figures from the various motions of the stars, their
'approaches', 'aspects' and 'conjunctions'. It was a prostitution and pretence of knowledge of events to come. He
bitterly regretted that he had formerly given himself up to it,
for he had come to know how erroneous and unfounded it was,
and how incompatible with reverence of God. He urged that the
understanding of 'days of crisis' was not in the least to be sought
in the shallow arguments of astrology, which contradict the well-
assured observations of the ancient physicians, and disturb the
sequence of the decretory days. It was true that formerly, deceived by the specious promises of astrological divination, and
not yet sufficiently versed in the practice of medical art, he had
thought otherwise. But what was really to be looked to was the
onset of the disease, its progress, the nature of the humour carrying the disease, and finally what is the usual course of Nature,
even though latent and occult, and the sympathy and harmony
of those days on which these steps occur; and the (patient's)
natural strength. By reflection on these points it might be possible
to foresee and predict the days on which in the conflict between
Nature and the malady, a rapid change would set in, whether
with favourable or fatal issue, or whether toward betterment or
the reverse. But the days of 'crisis' do not result from influences
of the stars and moon and their 'aspects', nor is dearth of the
humours brought about in that way, or tendency to crisis so
effected.[1]

In all this I am entirely at one with the teaching of this great
man. My view is that these impostors with their judicial astrology, pressing with extravagant zeal this absurd and ridiculous
view of the influence of the stars, outrage both heaven and
medicine. They are contemning the observations of the ancient
masters of medicine. Against the laws of Nature, they view
matter as taking exceptional and strange forms, and sublunar
bodies undergoing certain changes. They attribute these happenings to the 'aspects' and 'conjunctions' of the stars. They suppose
the physician will earn esteem and respect only if and in so far as
he shall foretell, from the motions, aspects and conjunctions of

1 Thevet's remark in the notice (1584) is that Fernel showed that
astronomy like antimony was to be used in medicine with moderation—
and never to be mixed up with prognosis.

the heavenly bodies, the calamities, conflagrations, plagues, wars, floods, epidemics and ills of every kind which afflict mankind; that it is by tracing such events, and their course, and divining their conclusion, that the physician has to arrive at an opinion. Nothing, to my mind, could be more untrue or absurd. I recognize willingly that often the Divine Power, whose decrees and plans are inscrutable, permits, in punishment of man's misdeeds, and in order to turn man back from his errors, pestilence and contagion, for him to bear. I will not deny even that the stars by their malignity corrupt the air to such a point that it becomes a source of mischief to man and beast, and sows the seeds of death. But I hold that none of these things can be foreseen by help of judicial astrology, and they are known only by their actual event. But to return to our theme.

His excusing himself from taking the office was accepted only on his feigning illness

Fernel, when unable to get permission from the dauphin to return to the capital, had to practise an imposition on him to obtain his sanction. He feigned pleurisy, and a surgeon in the prince's service undertook to tell the prince, that the physician was in grave danger, and that his illness was caused by sorrow and chafing at seeing himself withheld from his studies, separated from his wife and family, cut off from his lectures, forced to change his life of philosophic calm, study and peace, for the soldier's with its turmoil and its clamour; that he might succumb, if he could not return to his wife and his writing, his patients and his colleagues. To these arguments the dauphin yielded at last. He waived his opposition to Fernel's return to Paris. He ordered the honorarium which he had assigned to him still to be paid. He excused him from residing with the household, and from all irksome duties. He assured him he would make him his physician-in-chief, both for his skill in cure, and for his unique gift of prognosis. The gracious words of the prince soon drove away Fernel's feigned illness, and encouraged him more than ever to surmount the difficulties ahead.

After that he returned to his teaching of medicine

Two days after he got home, he took up again his interrupted treatise on blood-letting and sent it to the press. That task done, he thought of writing a commentary on certain parts of Hippocrates and Galen, as urged upon him daily by the candidates for the doctorate in medicine; they begged it of him, and complimented him. But the numbers of patients from all parts who came to him daily prevented his getting to the work.

He wrote the 'On the hidden causes of things'

Then indeed, that nothing of his time might pass undevoted to the good of the community, he spent his evenings writing a remarkable treatise 'On the hidden causes of things'. In it he dealt with the elements of all things, and especially with a number

of problems which are obscure in philosophy and medicine;
these in each case he treated so learnedly and appositely that he
is recognized as surpassing his contemporaries in this kind of
writing.

What impelled him to write the treatise was this. He felt that The reason
there are in the texts of the ancient philosophers and physicians for his
a number of statements which remain obscure and equivocal. writing it
With the help of some vague guessing each reader can make
these square with his opinion and twist them to his purpose.
Nevertheless the physician in the absence of some sure interpretation of them will feel himself at a loss for knowledge in important matters, and will be not rarely misled in the actual
practice of his calling. For definite settlement of these points,
as touched on in his physiological and other works, he thought
to give them a treatise to themselves, devoting detailed consideration to the controversial matters. He did so in order that
explanation of them might not interrupt, by digressions, frequently long, the course of the sustained argument, and break
the continuity of the subject in hand, and so tend to obscure what
was in itself clear.

A foundation, so to say, for medicine having thus been Pathology
supplied by these works, he finished in another few years a in seven
distinctive and remarkable treatise on disease, giving to it the books
title 'Pathology', and publishing it. He incorporated in it all
that is good, and that stands confirmed on a solid basis, in the
ancient writers, and added on his own account what he found
they had omitted. He removed uncertainties, cleared up obscurities, corrected mistakes, excised superfluities,[1] pinning himself
to no view given merely on authority alone, lest that involve him
in endorsing error.

It was his first object to teach how the signs of a disease can be On the com-
recognized with certainty, and, that done, how the disease is to pounding
be overcome. But in order not to disturb the continuity of the of drugs
description, by having to repeat after each separate disease how
to cure it, and the description of various sorts of medicaments,
he decided on an introductory explanation of medicaments,
simple and compound. In this, besides giving a number of new
compound ones, which his long experience knew to be extremely
valuable, and describing the way to employ them, he was at pains
to report also on those which were employed by the ancients,
and are kept by the apothecaries in their shops on daily demand.
He excluded all wholly foreign-grown stuff imported from

1 Here Plancy is following Fernel's own dedicatory Epistle to the King,
of 1554.

abroad, which is never to hand or only in a rotten state. He substituted for it home-grown products; and this was a real service to humanity.

Of all drugs he preferred the indigenous

It was his wont to say that the remedies native with us have a sort of affinity to ourselves, and that each part of the world has an ample stock of the medicaments proper for and particular to the complaints with which it is afflicted, remedies granted to it by the Author of Nature. He declared it was therefore a great mistake to extol and prescribe preferentially and almost exclusively medicaments which are exotic, brought from afar and consequently costly. He asserted that, since the French were the latest of all folk to take up medicine, a number of remedies which Nature produces within our own countryside, of use against the enemies of our own home side, to wit our home ailments, have still escaped our knowledge. These home-grown remedies are what call for active search; they should be brought into use and their names and virtues placed on record and kept in constant remembrance. So it is that, if he had not been cut off by untimely death, he would have been the most thorough investigator of our native remedies, purgatives, etc., and he would, at some time, have published a complete treatise on them.

After writing out the treatise on the composition of medicines he would read and re-read it. He was scrupulous in settling the right doses of the purgatives, and in examining their action on a number of individuals. He would not leave in his treatise any statement of their action which had not been ascertained by repeated trial.

Plancy gathered up the statements of the ancients on the virtues of the drugs and Fernel critically edited them

While he was engaged on this work on simples and their actions I got together, at his request, from the classical writers everything of importance they had to say on the subject. This I excerpted and collected for him. He subsequently examined it in detail and revised it. Against passages in it he would put the mark (·), which indicated that some day he would amplify it from experience of his own, that is, would describe, for the benefit of posterity, particular properties of the drug observed by himself, but missed by the ancients. He made the public cause and common weal a first charge on his learning and devotion; but nevertheless he was not willing that remedies, which arduous years of experience and practice of his own had found of striking and outstanding efficacy in difficult and obstinate disease, should forthwith be announced to all. He thought rather to keep them as a treasure and secret to himself, until his books, on being published, showed them to be of his own finding, and all would understand that they had been introduced first by himself, and thanks for them would be rendered to him by all. It is no new thing for even the noblest of men to be sensitive to fame, and fired by desire to promote his name's remembrance.

So it was that lest there should be wrested from him the fame and glory which were his, by right of many a wakeful and toil- some hour, he judged it best to delay the final touches to the treatise on simples and remedies, until he had ready for the press his work on the curing of diseases, with intent to publish them all at the same time.

He did not put the last touches

But, as a fact, while this was in his mind, the king, Henry of France, sought his counsel and upset all his plans. The king, on the death of his father, Francis, had succeeded to the throne. He summoned Fernel to take over the charge of the royal health. Henry had a lively regard for Fernel, on account of Fernel's rare learning and wonderful success in treatment; Henry (as dauphin) had already chosen him physician-in-chief to himself. Fernel's predilection for study, however, stood in the way of acceptance of the flattering offer. Very respectfully he submitted that on many grounds the appointment pertained almost of hereditary right to Maître de Bourges, physician-in-chief to the late King Francis, and that it was due to him. Fernel obtained leave from the king to prosecute, for the time being, amid his crowd of patients, his quest for yet more knowledge, and his enquiry into how his own observations agreed with the writings of the ancients, and his devising of new methods of treatment for still more difficult cases. But later on, when de Bourges died and his place had to be filled, Fernel could say no more.

because, although he had declined, he was once more

He was then about sixty years of age, but robust and inured to hard work. He felt that life at court, though strenuous, would not be more so than the laborious years he had spent in Paris, and survived. It seemed to him the court might indeed prove a welcome place of retreat in which to pursue his studies. His duties to the king and princes he might hope would leave him more leisure than was to be had in Paris, with all the calls upon him by the community. That expectation would certainly not have failed him, had not the war which France so long had waged with Spain and England, after a brief suspension, broken out again violently. The king, who always took Fernel with him, had to march with the army, now to one place now to another, bringing aid or developing support wherever the enemy gathered in force.

selected physician-in-chief to the king

However, amid all his preoccupations Fernel let no day pass without contributing a line to what he was writing. It was while he was on these journeys that he began to compose his treatise

At that
time he
wrote his
'Treatment
of fevers'

on the treatment of fevers,[1] and he was already almost through with it, when the king called him to accompany him, for the capturing of the sea-port Icium, called Calais, from the English who had occupied it for a hundred years.[2]

Then his
wife died

Returned thence Fernel joined the court at Fontainebleau, taking with him his wife. But she, accustomed to easy homely ways of life, pined under separation from her family, and after a few days developed a continued fever, which became extremely acute. Grievously prostrated by it, at length on the twentieth day of her illness she died delirious and convulsed.

Whence he
took fever
which
proved
early fatal

None of us can indeed be blessed in all ways. Fernel, who, in his not rare misfortunes, was, to my remembrance, never before thrown off his mental balance, maintaining his steadiness and courage, was now shrewdly hit by this loss of his wife. Indeed, he was overwhelmed. Torn with pain and sorrow he was, twelve days after the burial of his wife, himself taken ill with a continued fever.

History of
his fever:
first week

King Henry was in Paris at the time. On the news that Fernel had fever, and was already prostrate, he in his turn was deeply moved. He urged his other physicians to devote unsparing attention to Fernel, and to assure his recovery. He added: 'It would distress me beyond measure if he whom I have hardly ever thought myself likely to lose, should pass away.' So too the courtiers, and the foremost physicians, watched round Fernel, and did him common service. He, however, was not like those halting physicians, who, in the case of other people employ medical learning, but fail to treat themselves. On the contrary, he pondered over the fever he had contracted, and at once sought its primary cause, examined its character, and watched its least signs, in order to make a prognosis; in a word he was on the alert to trace everything which could throw light on his own case's nature and treatment. Then he proceeded to the preparation of the remedies which seemed best, and weighed with the physicians, who visited him daily, the opinions which were in agreement with his views.

Second
week

And, by Hercules, on the seventh day the urine cleared, and the febrile symptoms became less severe. The medical men in attendance anticipated a happy issue. But on the eleventh day all the symptoms became surprisingly severe. The sick man was struck by the bad state of the urine, and the violence of the other symptoms, and had apprehension that his case was fatal. He

1 Cf. Bibliog. 61.J5.
2 P. Bayle corrects to 211 years (*Dict. Historique et Critique*, vol. II, 1697).

called into consultation some of the best physicians of the court
and city.

As mentioned above, he had suffered from quartan fever, and
his custom always was to drink wine sparingly and much diluted
with water; and, between meals, in summer was wont to ease
his thirst with cooling drinks. Hence it was surmised that his
spleen might be not a little out of order. Moreover, there had
been for a whole two years a sensation of acidity in the mouth
and throat which treatment had not relieved. When therefore
to other grievous circumstances, the death of his wife added acute
distress, everything was aggravated further, and the humour,
gathered in the spleen, at length heating and decaying produced
an inflammation of that organ. So the continued fever was made
more severe and sensibly increased and wore out his natural
powers. Thus it was that premature death removed him from us,
on the eighteenth day of his illness, at the age of seventy-two,[1]
in the year of Our Lord 1557. Investigating by autopsy the cause
of his death we judged that the mischief had spread from an inflammation of the spleen, for that organ was markedly swollen
and was livid and greenish, and, when cut into by the scalpel, a
lot of sanious matter as black as pitch came from it.

On the fourteenth day of his illness, having little hope of recovery, Fernel became acutely troubled at the prospect of his
speedy decease. 'Not that I grieve to die', he said. 'I have
reached the term commonly set by Nature. I have attained fame.
My wife is gone before me; children I have. But for the sake of
learning and medicine I have not lived long enough.' To advance
these latter he had sacrificed all life's pleasures, and health itself.
What pained him especially was not to have put the finishing
touches to the therapeutical and last part of his *Medicina*. He had
long been busy upon it; it would have contained many discoveries
by him. As Pliny tells us Apelles left his 'Venus' unfinished and
in the rough, so Fernel had indeed not completed the final work
to which he had set his hand. All his undealt-with material he
devised to Guillaume Plancy, and Plancy will speak of it on
another occasion.

The news of the death of Jean Fernel came as a heavy sorrow
to the king, the queen and members of the court. It could not
but be so. The prince, humane and sympathetic, was deeply

Marginal notes:
Third week
and death

Therefore
was born
in 1485

He took
it as a heavy
blow

and the
king grieved

[1] Discrepancy between this and previous statement of age, *v. supra*,
p. 154. The Utrecht edition here omits the marginal in the original
edition (1607) which runs: 'LII forse scripsit, ita enim aevi clariss. nostri
historici et chronologi', meaning de Thou, who gives fifty-two as the
age of Fernel. *History of his own time*, bk. 21

moved by the loss of a renowned physician whose skill he had so often proved, and had watched with his eyes rescuing brave soldiers and illustrious captains, one whose hands had brought help to thousands. Nor did the great nobles mourn him less; for twenty years they had witnessed his success in their own serious illnesses and those of their retainers.

and indeed a loss to medicine

This man, less for the sake of himself than in truth for the community and for posterity, had toiled far into the night without remission or sparing of himself, because, with the host of sick resorting to him, he could not write during the day. His night's rest, short as it already was, he cut shorter and at severe cost to his own health. In elucidating physiology and pathology he had shown himself easily superior to all other writers of the century. What may we not suppose he would have done, practising in Paris, the admired and praised of all, with a host of patients, if the Fates had allowed him to enlighten with his discoveries the therapeutical part of medicine. But that is the uncertainty hanging over poor mortals, and none can attain wholly the supreme height or accomplish his desire.

Struggles he had had in his life

When he began practice in Paris, certain learned physicians, already high in favour, tried to block his way and to check him at the beginning of his career. But before long, I know not by what fatality, death cut them off before their time; Fernel, freed from that rivalry, soon outdistanced the rest.

with Flexelle

A certain one there was, named Flexelle,[1] who at a time when he was already well known and respected by the town plotted to upset and suppress him. Since he and Fernel aimed at the very height and top of all that pertains to the sacred calling of medicine, and each felt himself a leader in his art, there was in the struggle between them little room for mutual appreciation. Flexelle, eager for fame, and spurred by jealousy, watched Fernel, whom he could not accuse of ill-will or ignorance or discourtesy, outdistance the other physicians of the town, men older than himself and, before his arrival, high in popular favour. Fernel surpassed him both in earnestness and repute; Flexelle obstructed Fernel's efforts and schemed to rob him of his reputation and put an end to his fame.

1 Goulin (*Mémoires*, p. 517) supplies some information about Flexelle. He seems to have engaged chiefly in surgery. Ambroise Paré relates an incident which, as Goulin remarks, indicates that Flexelle was an impetuous and coarse character. He wrote a small Introduction to Surgery, Goulin thinks in french. He was a physician to Francis I, Henri II, Francis II and Charles IX. He took his M.D. two years before Fernel. Goulin says of him 'il veut réussir *per fas et nefas*'.

A handle which could be used for this purpose was the follow- How it
ing. In cacochymia, even when accompanied by plethora, Fernel arose
was against lavish letting of blood. He was content with
purgation for drawing off the humour to which the disease was
due. Now, to bleed is to withdraw all the humours together,
often with shock to the patient's strength, and especially mis-
chievously when the cacochymia is due to obstruction of the
liver or mesentery or lack of innate heat or from weakness of the
stomach (which is frequent enough), as in some kinds of jaundice,
and in cachexias and leucophlegma. Flexelle, on the other hand,
ordered copious and frequent blood-letting in all fevers caused
by a putrid humour, as well as in many other diseases due to
cacochymia, even when not associated with plethora.

We see that both of them carried their views too far. Fernel Was it
employed bleeding too sparingly, too carefully, and sometimes satisfactory?
not at all, when he should have bled. On the contrary Flexelle
employed it too often and immoderately, in almost every ailment, alike whether of cold or febrile type, and against the advice
of other physicians. And we ourselves have often seen the patient
in consequence prostrated and wasted, the 'spirits' and the innate
heat spent, so that rapid death, or dropsy, or some other grave
and perilous condition supervened.

Now, Flexelle dared not attack Fernel in writing, or by public His correct
disputation in the Schools. He adopted the mean course of de- attitude won
faming him behind his back. Fernel's disregard of these attacks through
made Flexelle furious. He did not scruple to speak of the man
who, by his public lectures and by the treatises he had produced,
had demonstrated his exceptional knowledge to the whole world,
as an ignorant fellow, an impostor and a charlatan. Fernel, however, never permitted himself any abuse of Flexelle nor, although
attacked, did he hit back. He spoke no ill of him nor sought to
detract from his reputation. If at any time someone told him of
Flexelle's attacks upon him, he would hope for him a better
frame of mind in the future. But whenever called to a patient
along with Flexelle he declined the case, saying he had other
pressing business, or was on a holiday.

Fernel was unpopular with not a few of his profession, indeed His relations
he was, one may say, hated. For one thing, he did not allow the with others
medicines he prescribed for those of his patients who were
dangerously ill to be sent as was customary to the apothecaries;
he either prepared them himself at his house, or entrusted them
to a few friends on whom he could rely. I am not aware, however, that this has been considered reprehensible in anyone
hitherto.

Fernel's way
of life

But of this enough. Let me now devote a few words to the manner in which practice was carried on in Paris at the time when Fernel began there.

Inspection of
urine and
work before
dinner

In France the old-established custom was for people of the commoner sort, when they fell ill, to send the urine forthwith to a physician. He would discover from it not only how long the patient had been ill, and of what kind the illness was, and what part was particularly affected, and what the especially troublesome symptoms were, but also the patient's sex and age. It had already long been a practice for certain rascally impostors and empirics, falsely and with brazen impertinence, to take to themselves the name and dignity of 'physician' and to advertise to the public their skill in this. Indeed they would declare that the physician who could not from inspection of the urine follow all diseased conditions of the body, and even disturbances of the mind, was unworthy of the title of physician. It was from the purlieus of such as these that there issued those famous books, of incomparable (save the mark) service to the public, treating of prognostication from the urine, tomes whose crude rules the physician, in his novitiate, is still taught, twisted labyrinths of empty words, for deluding the minds and judgement of those who bring to them the urine—a confused list, an impudent hotchpotch of symptoms, so that if perchance the sick person complained of a single one of the items in it, the list would have hit off the case. It would then be supposed that the interpretation had been correct, and the whole history of the case been understood from the urine.

So indeed it came about that Fernel, following custom, accepted this common practice of physicians, wrong and debased though we must admit it was. At the outset of his practice he made inspection of urines. Rising at about 4 o'clock every morning he went from his bedroom down to his library. There he looked over some page of text of the ancient masters, either because he did not feel satisfied about it, or that he did not sufficiently remember it, or in order to add to it something by way of commentary. After that, with the coming of daylight, he went out to his public lectures, or to visit his patients. Then it was that urines were brought to him and he would inspect them. What he opined about them he made known, and ordered treatment according to the cause of the disease, and the constitution of the patient, as far as he could gather those by conjecture.

Dinner and
supper

Back again for his meal, he retired to his library while dinner was being prepared, and when dinner was over retired thither again, until the time for resuming his 'visits'. It was the same

before supper while the table was being got ready. After supper
he returned to his study and did not finally retire until
11 o'clock, by which time heaviness came on, and drove him to
go up to sleep. This was his way of work and life for more than
thirty years. Through all that time he kept up this programme
of study. Amusement, whether of body or mind, he held as
nothing in comparison with the study and practice of the art of
medicine. There was no hour of his life which was not given
to duty private or public, professional or domestic. If perchance
he invited a guest to sup or to dine, he did not consider it wrong
or discourteous to excuse himself soon after the meal, for the
sake of his studies.

His wife had persuaded him, some years before his death, to
buy a country house at Pantin, whither he could withdraw at
times, as to a tranquil haven, for recruitment after the turmoil
of the restless city. As a fact it was hardly once or twice in the
year that he cared to go there. The robust disposition of his mind,
and its inclination toward fortitude and ·duty, made him averse
to all relaxation. He consecrated the whole course of his life to
effort, bodily and mental. No rest, no relaxation, no social entertainments afforded him pleasure, nor the pursuits of his contemporaries nor their amusements. He thought nothing in life
worth while except that which should count toward honour and
glory and high desert. Of all that engages mankind, there was
nothing in his view finer or greater than good service to the
christian commonwealth, to succour the suffering, to free the
sick from their danger, to promote the health of all, to consider
his own health only after that of the community, and finally
to avert disease by shutting all its avenues of access. The
number of those who came to consult him became so large
that, almost the summer through, he had to take his dinner
without even sitting down. He let no one, however poor, go away
without information as to the disease from which he suffered,
and unprovided with a remedy for its treatment. When occa-
sionally I warned him to take more care of his health, to intermit
his nightly vigil, and begged him to get more rest (for he allowed
himself only a minimum of sleep), he was wont to have this reply
ready: 'Fate will grant us a long repose' (*Longa quiescendi tempora
fata dabunt*).

His face was thoughtful, severe and sad, but it wore a smile
and became gracious when he approached a sick person. He
questioned them kindly and sympathetically about the slightest
symptom, as he tried to discover the cause of the illness and what
might be the part affected. I doubt if in any disease he ever met,
however obscure, he failed to recognize its source and character.

Marginal notes:

His country house and relaxation

His manner with the patient

170   *APPENDIX*

Were it never so complex, never so strange, he soon referred it
to its class, and traced its origins, such was his gift of penetrative
insight, and his clearness of thought and judgement.

In hopeless diseases Never did he discourage even those at the door of death, and
those already wept over as doomed; he held out hope of recovery
always. In cases where the turn the illness might take was not
yet clear, he used to wrap his prognosis in ambiguous words
which others might repeat or interpret either way. He could
hardly be induced at the outset of an illness to speak of what the
event might be, and he would expressly explain that such prediction as he ventured was in the nature of a guess. For chronic
illnesses his prognosis was scarcely ever wrong. In pronouncing,
in answer to afflicted friends, that a fatal issue was to be feared,
his countenance grew overcast and gloomy, and his voice became
dolorous and high-pitched; but when he could predict the recovery of the patient, his face would light up and his tone of voice
convey his gladness. He never encouraged ill stories about other
physicians; he felt the like might some day be directed against
himself, and physicians of merit.

After the medicine had been prescribed When he was called to visit a man of parts, after he had
diagnosed and prescribed, he liked—time and the state of the case
permitting—to enter into talk with him; with a philosopher on
philosophy, with a mathematician on mathematics, with a
commander or soldier on the sites of towns, the rivers on which
they stand, or engines of war and their inventors, with a sailor
on navigation and newly discovered lands, with a theologian on
God and the things of heaven, with a business man on commerce.
In these talks he would contrive, as occasion offered, to bring
forward some comforting assurance, and fortify the patient's
hopes. And he would relieve a serious theme with touches of
humour to lighten it. All this gained him respect and liking from
everyone, so that he was esteemed a man of geniality and wit.

The sort of man he was bodily Fernel was fairly tall, and his constitution was robust, but he
had been weakened by violent attacks of renal pain recurring
four and five times a year. His complexion was dark and sallow;
his hair was very black and thick.

Mentally As for the character of his mind, when anger seized him he
repressed it swiftly. Habitually preoccupied with his own
thoughts, he was rather sad and taciturn. He told no one his
plans, and was mistrustful in most ways. He supervised his
household affairs carefully, but that did not prevent his being a
liberal and generous friend.

How much his practice brought him Throughout the time I lived with him (and I lived with him
for ten years) his annual income often exceeded twelve thousand
French pounds and rarely fell below ten.

NOTE III. CLICHTOVEUS (p. 9)

JOSSÉ CLICHTOWE (1472–1543, at Chartres) studied at Paris and took the Doctor's degree in 1506. He was from Niewpoort, in the Netherlands. He collaborated with Lefèvre d'Étaples in text-books and commentaries on Aristotle and Boethius. Lefèvre's Commentary on Aristotle's *Physics* and the *Parva Naturalia* is said to have actually changed the treatment of natural science in the University of Paris. Clichtowe's own works indicate the trend toward humanism. He developed ideas of the state gathered from the classics.[1] In his 'On War and Peace'[2] he discussed the ethics of war and defended a pacific attitude. He also wrote justifying the worship of certain of the Saints.[3] His tractate 'On True Nobility' was translated into the vernacular (1529). He was of course much senior to Fernel at the University, and of an altogether older generation than Plancy: for the latter's attitude toward him, cf. the text.

NOTE IV. '*INSIDIOSÆ PACIS*' (p. 10)

ON the title-page Bened. Rigaud the publisher has his mark and motto 'Pietate et Justicia' (in the form which Baudrier numbers 25 and figures, ser. iii, p. 459). Consists of 8 pp., 8°, italic character. The only copy cited by Baudrier is in the Lyons Biblioth. At end of the poem, after *Finis*, is 'Deo gloria et gratia' (? the author's motto). The address given by the colophon is a Paris one (though not mentioned as such). It is that of Phil. Pigouchet, printing 1488–1516, who was succeeded by Pierre Attaignant, who died not later than 1553. Attaignant was the earliest in Paris to print music from movable type. He married the daughter of Pigouchet, and after his death his widow succeeded him in the business. Bened. Rigaud was for a number of years the government printer at Lyons, issuing royal decrees, arrêts, etc. He was so at the time of publishing this poem. His business aimed at publishing poetry, French history, modern law and medicine, at low prices; the products of his press suffered in consequence somewhat in quality (paper and workmanship), but are nevertheless much sought by collectors. Baudrier states of him, 'he was equally opposed to the excesses of the Catholic League and to the violences of the huguenots'. In 1573 he published the *Généalogie et la Fin des Huguenaux, & descouverte du Calvinisme*, par M. Gabriel de Saconay, 8°, with pictures.

1 *De Regis Officio opusculum, quid optimum quemque regem deceat* (On the scope of Kingship and what best becomes every King), Paris, Henri Estienne, 30 August 1519, 4°, 72 ff.

2 *De Bello et Pace opusculum, Christianos Principes ad sedandos Bellorum Tumultus et Pacem componendam exhortans*, Paris, S. de Colines, 1523, 4°, 52 ff.

3 *De laudibus S. Ludovici Regis Franciae; de Laudibus Martyris Ceciliae*, Paris, Henri Estienne, 10 January, 1516, 4°, 66 ff.

NOTE V. JACQUES GOVEA (p. 14)

JACQUES GOVEA, whom Fernel addresses as 'mathematician', and to whom he inscribes his first book, was of a Portuguese family, more than one member of which attained eminence in France. In due course Jacques became Rector of Ste Barbe, at that time a headquarters of the Portuguese and Spanish students frequenting Paris. The Collège de Ste Barbe received Francis Xavier in 1525, and in 1528 Ignatius Loyola, already a man of thirty-five, both of them students from the Spanish Basque country. Xavier was appointed lecturer on Aristotle in 1528. Fernel, if we follow Goulin's chronology for him, was lecturing on Aristotle there at the same time, and residing in the College. The tone of Fernel's dedication of his book to Govea is warm enough to denote affection as well as respect. Similarly, the relation between Govea and Loyola is known to have amounted to deep and life-long personal attachment.[1] Loyola, already in ripe manhood, had put himself to College to learn latin and then philosophy. But he was vowed to poverty, and had surrendered all his goods. He was thus at the mercy of students who were, in the main, 'overgrown boys', and did not for a time understand his asceticism. Govea, when he came to know him, had sheltered and befriended him in the College. It was in that 'warm nest', as Fernel called it, and at that very time, that Fernel was busied with his three early 'philosophical' books. It must have been a society embracing Govea, Loyola, Xavier and Fernel, each early in his career. Celaya, the Thomist, e.g. 'Porphyry', 1516, went home to Spain in 1525.

NOTE VI. GOULIN'S RESEARCHES REGARDING FERNEL (p. 16)

JEAN GOULIN held the Chair of Medical History in the Paris Faculty from 1795 to 1799. In 1775 he published (Paris) a quarto volume *Mémoires littéraires, critiques philologiques, biographiques et bibliographiques pour servir à l'histoire ancienne et moderne de la Médecine*. Dédiés à Monseigneur la Garde des Sceaux, Louis XVI régnant.[2] In its Preface he mentions that the book has occupied him for fifteen years. Among its contents is a translation, with notes, of Plancy's 'Life' of Fernel. The translation is followed by two historical appendices and a bibliography of Fernel's works.

1 *Ignatii Loiolae Vita*, auctore Joanne Petro Maffeio, Barcelone, typis Huberti Gutandi, 1589, bk. i, cc. 19 and 20. Also, *Vida. Virtudes y Miliagros de S. Ignacio de Loyola*, por el padre Francisco Garcia, de la misma Compañia, Madrid, 1685, bk. ii, c. 12, pp. 151-8.

2 No author's name appears on the title. The name is only found as signature to the dedicatory letter, and there without a fore-name. Besides the *Mémoires* Goulin published *Lettres à un Médecin de province sur l'histoire de la Médecine*, 1769, Paris.

Goulin seems to have been a character at once austere and quaint —an 'oddling' in Ben Jonson's sense. An account of him and of his literary work, by Citizen P. Sue,[1] was issued the year after his death, 'an VIII' of the Republic. Sue was professor and librarian at the École de Médecine, Paris, where Goulin had been professor of the History of Medicine. Much of Goulin's life had been a struggle against a poverty which thwarted his pursuits as a scholar. His father died early and his mother pinched herself to provide education for the boy. He did well at school, and then for a time earned a living as a teacher at a salary of 100 francs a year, and, even so, was often out of work. He wrote of himself that 'in some years he had no more resources than a beggar in the streets'. He scraped together means to pursue in Paris the courses on medicine. In season and out of season he prosecuted his researches into ancient texts and inscriptions. In 1766 he earned a competence for the first time. His biographer says of him that if, in quest of the best rendering of a greek or latin passage, he had been for some time without finding one to his taste, he would go to bed, even at midday, and there remain for one, two or even three days, except for a meal and sleep, lost in reflection. In that way the suitable interpretation would offer itself at last. His room was never tidy—disorder reigned, except in his ideas and his books—these latter always accumulating. The Librarian of the Bibliothèque Nationale called him the 'Bienfaiteur', because he presented to the National Library a number of unprocurable books, despite his very modest means. He was a man of punctilious probity. In his political views he was a convinced republican.

Goulin's painstaking enquiries seem to establish that Fernel was born in 1497. Plancy's 'Life', as it comes down to us, states that when Fernel died in 1557 (o.s.; in our reckoning 1558) he was seventy-two. Plancy nowhere gives the year of his birth. The marginals inserted in the Utrecht edition (1656) by the Heurnes state (twice over) '1485' as the year of Fernel's birth. But the Heurnes have omitted the marginal given in the original edition (1607), which says that according to the historian (de Thou) Fernel died at the age of fifty-two—not seventy-two. Goulin's estimate would make him sixty-two. Thevet's account gives his age as seventy-two; Pascal Gallus, as forty-nine. On various counts Goulin's statement appears the right one.

On certain points Goulin's references to Fernel seem in error. Thus:

1. *The date of the 'Cosmotheoria.'* Goulin gives it as 1529, and after *De Proportionibus*: but it seems to have been before the *De Proportionibus* and of date 1528 (see Appendix: bibliographical list).

---

1 *Mémoire historique, littéraire, et critique sur la Vie et sur les Ouvrages tant imprimés que manuscrits de Jean Goulin, Professeur de l'Histoire de la Médecine, à l'École de Médecine de Paris,* 8°.

174 APPENDIX

2. *Fernel's acquaintance with greek.* There is in Plancy's 'Life' a sentence which, after mention of the pleasure Fernel got from Celsus, refers to his reading Plato, and adds that Plato had recently been translated by Marsilio Ficino. Goulin infers (p. 293, footnote) from this that Fernel did not himself read greek. Figard (p. 17) repeats this, following Goulin. But: (1) Plancy, in the dedication of his *Galen's Commentary on Hippocrates' Aphorisms* to Fernel, says explicitly of Fernel that he read greek. His words are: 'Tibi vero, docte Ferneli, hanc ingenii nostri foeturam nuncupare visum est, non quod ea aut ad nominis celebritatem (es enim libris editis clarissimus) aut ad lectionem, qui Graecè calles et Graeca legere mavis (you who are versed in greek and prefer to read the greek); sed quia et ex ea ratione qua praeceptori discipulus debet aliquid, et privatim etiam aliis nominibus me tibi obligatum esse sciam; tum etiam ut si fortè labor noster tibi probabitur, fructum ipsius amplissimum cepisse me putem'.[1] 'Our production' and 'our work' possibly refer to the content of the annotations. (2) Fernel is accustomed to explain the meaning he attaches to a latin word or phrase used technically by giving a greek equivalent, e.g. αἱμάτωσις for 'generatio sanguinis' in the liver. In the *Medicina* of 1554, after the fourth book of the 'Pathology' he attaches to the latin text greek marginalia regularly. (3) In the 'Dialogue' (bk. ii, c. 6) he quotes passages from Galen[2] in greek. He would hardly have done these things had he not known greek.

3. *Date of writing of the 'Dialogue' (De Abditis Rerum Causis).* Goulin was unaware that the 'Dialogue' had been in existence, and probably circulated, before the first appearance of the 'Physiology', *De naturali parte Medicinae* (1542). He says expressly he has not been able to see a copy of the 1542 edition, and does not know of one. In that first edition, however, references are given to the 'Dialogue', showing that, before the printing of the 'Dialogue' by Wechel, in 1548, it had, presumably in MS., been, at least limitedly, accessible. These same marginal references to the 'Dialogue' are also in the second edition of the *De naturali parte Medicinae* (1547), Venice, and the 'Dialogue' is mentioned as an item in the Index. It seems that the earliest issue of the *De naturali parte Medicinae* to which Goulin had access was that of Lyons, 1551. The references establishing the prior existence of the 'Dialogue' are four, and occur:

(1) In bk. ii, c. 8, where the text runs: 'Cujus opinionis levitas alio loco a nobis refutata, fusiorē hic disputationem non desiderat.' The 'refutation in another place' refers to 'Dialogue', bk. i, c. 2. There it is suggestive that the 'Dialogue', although furnished with many marginal references, has

1 *Galeni in Aphorismos Hippocratis Commentarii*, VII. Recens per Gulielmum Plantium Cenomanum Latinitate donati ejusdemque annotationibus illustrati. Lyons, Guill. Rouille, 1552, 8°, 1st edit. Dedicat. to 'Joanni Fernelio, medico eximio'.
2 *Liber de foetus formatione.*

none to this discussion in the *De naturali parte Medicinae* printed six years earlier. That is to say, the book printed earlier gives a reference to the one as yet unprinted, while the book printed later gives no reference to the same subject in the book printed earlier. This would be accounted for by the later printed being the earlier written, and then being printed unaltered as written.

(2) In bk. iii, c. 2: 'In illa formarum remissione quātum sit lapsus, perpēsum à nobis alio loco est.' A marginal is supplied: 'dialogorū lib. 1'. In the edition of 1547 (Venice) this mention of the 'Dialogue' is listed as an item in the Index as follows: 'Dialogorum, Joan. Ferne. lib. 1.'

(3) In bk. iv, c. 1: 'Quare necesse est hūc vitę calorem praestantioris cujusdam esse originis, neque ignei elementi rudiorem naturam redolere, quemadmodum alio loco uberiùs disputatum est à nobis.' A marginal is supplied and runs: 'Primo Dialog. Calori nostro non opponitur frigus.'

(4) In bk. v, c. 17 (becomes c. 18 in editions of 1554 and later): 'Inest tum igitur ceu illius pars duntaxat et quaedam facultas, quemadmodum quae in osse, aut que in carne est forma quum iam totius species appulerit, supererit quidem non re ipsa et energia, sed tanquam praeparatio et facultas ministra formae succedentis, quod plenius alio loco disputavimus.' The marginal here says: 'Lib. 1 dialog.' Oddly, the translator of 1655, and Figard (p. 347) translating into french this passage in his 'Fernel' of 1903, both turn the past tense 'disputavimus' into the future—'discuterai'. This, of course, destroys the passage as an indication that the 'Dialogue' was written before the 'Physiology'. The translation (by Charles de Saint-Germain, doctor of the Faculty of Medicine, councillor and physician-in-ordinary to the king) of 1655 gives no marginals. But the marginal of the original has been noticed and its reference supposed to be to a 'Dialogue' by Aristotle. Thus, in view of the marginal in bk. iv, c. 1 of the 'Physiology', he introduces into the text there 'de la vient qu'Aristote au I des Dialogues, porte etc.' The edition of the 'Physiology' used was of 1554 or later.

4. *Fernel and the sterility of Catherine de Medici.* A statement, often made, that Fernel cured the sterility of Queen Catherine, is examined at considerable length by Goulin. He comes to the conclusion that there is no 'authentic proof of this brilliant cure'. He is writing in 1775. It is a little difficult to conceive what kind of proof he would expect. But he goes with fullness into documents *pro* and *con*. He stresses, as evidence of the weakness of the claim, that the opinion cannot be traced back farther than Scévole de Ste Marthe's *éloge* of Fernel published in the 1607 edition of Fernel's *Universa Medicina*. The statement, he points out, is 'forty years after the death of Fernel'. The words are 'invisam sterilitatem à domo regiâ repelleret'. But J. Sambucus, in his *Icones* of 1574 (Plantin, Antwerp), which give a portrait of Fernel, writes 'Sterilitatem à domo regiâ repulit, Valesium nomen optatâ generosae probis accessione propagandum curavit',

and that was nearly thirty years earlier than Scévole de Ste Marthe, and within sixteen years of Fernel's death, and cf. Thevet in 1583.

Goulin argues that, if Fernel had cured the queen's 'sterility', Plancy would have said so in the 'Life'. But several things which might appear likely to be mentioned by Plancy's 'Life' are not found there. There is no mention of Plancy's dedication of his Hippocrates or of Fernel's part in the annotating; no mention of two important treatises left complete but unpublished at Fernel's death, and entrusted to Plancy, and no mention, by name, of Fernel's first three works published in folio by de Colines. Of course, the 'Life' as it appeared is very brief; Wechel may have cut out parts of the original.

Again, the attribution to Fernel of the cure of the queen's 'sterility' occurs in some lines in the 1638 edition of the *Pathologia*, dedicated to Guy Patin. They are latin elegiacs signed 'N. Borbonius'.

De Operibus Joannis Fernelii Admirandae doctrinae medici Epigramma

Is simul ac francae medicus successerat aulae,
    Crevit felici regia prole nurus,
Viscera faecundat cui pigra, potentibus herbis
    Atque uteri segnes increpat arte moras;
Desperata prius tumuerunt pondera ventris,
    Mater et è sterili mox numerosa fuit:
Ante diu fueras casura Valesia proles,
    Pignora nî MEDICE tot medicata daret.
Ergo uterum potuit qui sollicitare morantem,
    Naturae clausas et reserare vias,
An dubites, (haec si satis intellecta legentur)
    Fecerit ut nasci, quin vetat ille mori?

Goulin, discussing these lines, writes: 'It is certainly not of himself' (i.e. spontaneously) 'that Nicolas Bourbon here praises Fernel for having put an end to the sterility of Catherine de Medici. He has done it at the request of Guy Patin and on the word of Ste Marthe.' 'Nicolas Bourbon was not born when Francis II' (Catherine's first-born) 'came into the world. Nicolas Bourbon was born in 1574, that is sixteen years after the death of Fernel.' Goulin does not allude to a possibility that the lines were by the elder Nicolas Bourbon (1503–1550), who wrote latin poems, some of them addressed to Henri II. In his small volumes, published in Paris by his friend Michael Vascosan, 1547 and 1549, four poems have 'Henry of Valois' as their subject, not to include a fifth addressed to him along with his father, the late King. But there are no verses on Fernel. Patin's 'Borboniana' has nothing to the point.

The upshot of the evidence would seem to be that the removal of Catherine's sterility was put to the credit of her physician, Fernel, by popular opinion at the time, and was part of his fame after his death.

5. *Catherine de Medici and Astrology.* In a note to Plancy's 'Life' of Fernel, Goulin declares Catherine de Medici 'little addicted to astrology'. But when Henri II visited the session of Parliament in Paris in 1558, the year of Fernel's death, and heard the complaints addressed to him by representative members, Anne de Bourg and others, one of the protests made to him concerned the astrological practices prevalent at the court. Henri himself was not enthusiastic about astrology. The inference is that the protest referred to the queen.

Catherine, with her Florentine connections and the influence there of Ficino, the neo-Platonist, who drew horoscopes for the Medici children, certainly listened to astrological prediction. De Thou's *History* (bk. xxii) states that Catherine consulted a 'mathematician' on the fates of her husband and sons. When Nostradamus, the notorious astrologer-physician, visited the court and drew up the astrological predictions on Catherine's children, it was at her—not at the king's—instance. Also she received from Spanish sources reports of astrological and magical procedures intended to work mischief on the heads of the Reformed Church party. Her library is known to have been rich in books on astrology.

NOTE VII. SHELLFISH AND THE MOON (p. 36)

THE reputed phenomenon around which this belief centres was mentioned by Aristotle.[1] It was the subject of a proposal, put forward in the early days of the Royal Society (*Phil. Trans. London*, ii, 1667), that travellers in the East Indies should enquire 'whether those shellfishes, that are in these parts plump and in season at the full moon, and lean and out of season at the new, are found to have contrary constitutions in the East Indies'.[2] An answer was obtained in 1923 by Professor H. Munro Fox, F.R.S. (*Proc. Roy. Soc. B*, xcv, pp. 523–50). 'At Suez,' he writes, 'sea-urchins and crabs are said to be "full" at full moon and "empty" at new moon, at Alexandria the same thing is said of mussels and of sea-urchins; the Tarentines believe that oysters are fattest at full moon, while at Nice, Naples, Alexandria, and in Greece urchins are said to be fullest at full moon.' 'My own investigations have shown that while the supposition is untrue of mussels (*Mytilus* sp.) and sea-urchins (*Strongylocentrotus lividus*) in the Mediterranean, and of mussels (*Mytilus variabilis*) and crabs (*Neptunus pelagicus*) in the Red Sea, it is based on fact as concerns the sea-urchins

1 Also Pliny, *Natural History*, ii, 102, trans. by Bostock and Riley, London, 1855.
2 A reply received from Sir Philibert Vernatti, resident in Batavia, is given by Bishop Sprat, *Hist. of the Roy. Soc.* 1667, p. 161. It runs: 'I find it so here, by experience in Batavia, in oysters and crabs.'

found at Suez (*Centrechinus* (*Diadema*) *setosus*). In the last-mentioned form the gonads undergo a cycle of growth and development corresponding with each lunation throughout the breeding season. Just before full moon ovaries and testes are at their greatest bulk, filled with spermatozoa or eggs which are spawned into the sea at the time of full moon. The shrunken gonads then gradually fill again with ripening sexual products, to be shed at the next full moon. It is remarkable, then, that a belief, which was such common knowledge among the ancient inhabitants of Mediterranean countries that it was referred to by their poets and orators, and one which is held to-day in the Mediterranean ports, is indeed untrue of this region, while at Suez it is based on fact. It is possible that the Greeks originally obtained the belief from the ancient Egyptians, who would have it from the Red Sea (what really occurs there in sea-urchins being supposed to apply to all "shellfish"), and that the same belief has survived around the Mediterranean until to-day.'

NOTE VIII. VALCHER'S TRACTATES (p. 38)

VALCHER's volume shows the University of Padua still 'Arab' at the end of the sixteenth century. It offers some interest aside from the medical text. The dedication of the 'Variola' treatise is to a noble Venetian, Aloisius Pisaurius. It recalls how 'it must be now some twelve years since first my odd fortune led me to Venice and to your friendship. The latter I cannot claim to have ground for in myself; its ground lay simply in your great kindness to a student following philosophy. I remember how friendlily and freely you received me, a young man and a stranger unknown to you, and unfurnished with a recommendation from anyone at all. It was just because you understood me to be someone engaged in following philosophy. You introduced me to your illustrious friends.' The letter goes on to mention them by name. The prefatory letter of the other dissertation, also written at Padua and in the same month, relates that an outbreak of the plague and other misadventures were what had brought Valcher (? Walker) first to Padua, and that he had found there a seat of learning which, 'while paying no less attention than do Oxford and Cambridge to the three languages, left them far behind in its pursuit of the treasures of philosophy and medicine'. He mentions that he had before coming to Padua spent five years at Oxford. The person to whom this dedication is addressed is an Englishman then in Venice—'Rev^mus Dom. D. Ricardus Scelleius, Meletensis Militiae in Anglia Praefectus, et primus ejus Regni Baro'—namely, Sir Richard Shelley, the last Grand Prior of the Knights of Malta in England. A condensed account of Sir Richard Shelley's varied and travelled life is given in the *Dictionary of National Biography* (A. F. Pollard). Of a Sussex family—that family whence later came the poet Shelley— active against the Reformation, he was always under suspicion from the

Protestants. In 1539 he accompanied the Venetian Ambassador to Constantinople. He is said to have been the first Englishman to visit that city after its capture by the Turks. In 1555 he was commissioned to carry to the King of Portugal the news of the expectation of the birth of a child to Mary of England. When Mary re-established in England the Order of St John, Sir Richard was made 'turco-polier' of the Order, i.e. appointed to the command of the light troops. He was in Malta immediately after the great siege, and was then made Grand Prior of the Order, but in deference to the wishes of Queen Elizabeth, he did not use the title. When Valcher dedicated to him this treatise, on 'Variola', Shelley was, at the express invitation of the Seignory of Venice, residing in Venice, where he was treated with distinction. He died there about the year 1589.

NOTE IX. LIST OF J. RIOLAN THE ELDER'S WORKS ON FERNEL (p. 44)

1. *Ad librum Fernelii de Spiritu et calido innato Jo. Riolani commentarius.* Paris, at T. Brumennius, 1570, 8°, 16 ff.
2. *Ad librum Fernelii de Elementis Joannis Riolani commentarius.* Paris, at T. Brumennius, 1575, 8°, 12 ff.
3. *Ad librum Fernelii de Temperamentis Joannis Riolani commentarius.* Paris, at T. Brumennius, 1576, 8°, 16 ff.
4. *Ad_librum Fernelii de Facultatibus animae Joannis Riolani commentarius. Inserta est disputatio philosophica de immortalitate animi.* Paris, at T. Brumennius, 1577, 8°.
5. *Ad librum Fernelii de Procreatione hominis Jo. Riolani commentarius.* Paris, at T. Brumennius, 1578, 8°, 20 ff.
6. *Joannis Riolani in Libros Fernelii partim Physiologicos, partim Therapeuticos Commentarii. Accesserunt ejusdem Riolani, De primis principiis rerum naturalium,* Lib. III. Mompelgarti (Montbéliard), at Jacob Foyllet, 1588, 8°, 480 pp.
7. *Ad libros Fernelii de abditis rerum causis J. Riolani commentarius.* Paris, at H. Perier, 1598, 12°, prelim. + 165 pp.
8. ...... (Paris, 1602), 8°.
9. *J. Riolani Praelectiones in libros physiologicos, et de abditis rerum caussis* (sic) *cum brevibus scholiis.* Paris, by H. Perier ex officio Plantin, 1601, 8°, 4 parts in 2 vols.
10. *Universae medicinae compendia per Joannem Riolanum.* Paris, by H. Perier, ex officio Plantiniana, 1598, 8°, 178 ff.
11. ...... 1606, 8°, 3rd edit., 172 ff.
12. ...... 1618, 8°, 4th edit., 340 pp. + index.
13. *Universae medicinae compendium auctore Joanne Riolano.* Paris, by S. Perier, 1626, 12°, index + 348 pp.

NOTE X.   THE FATAL TOURNEY-WOUND
OF HENRI II OF FRANCE (p. 54)

HENRI died from a wound accidentally inflicted in the tourneys held at
Paris in July 1559. He had asked a gentleman of the Guard, Montgomery,
to repeat an encounter with him. Montgomery's lance splintered and, by
misadventure, penetrated Henri's eye and brain. He died ten days
later, after great suffering relieved by spells of unconsciousness. He insistently exonerated Montgomery from all blame. There are contemporary
prints of the scene at the tournament, and of Paré and Vesalius at the bedside of Henri, in a volume, printed at Geneva, 1569 [engravers *Tortorel
et Périssin*] (folio), by Nicol Castellin de Tournai. The book is 'the first
part'; but no further part was issued.

Montgomery, of the fatal tournament, was Count Gabriel de Montgomery, Captain of the Scots Guard. He embraced the Huguenot cause
later, and became a notable Huguenot commander. He was at one time
condemned to death by the Parlement de Paris, and was executed in
effigy. He narrowly escaped the massacre of St Bartholomew, being
pursued by the Guises more than twenty miles. Finally, fighting in Nor-
mandy, in 1574, he was forced to surrender to superior forces. The terms
of surrender spared his life. But later he was executed under orders from
the Queen-Regent, Catherine de Medici. It was rumoured she had not
forgotten the fatal tournament. But on this compare *Le Discours Merveil-
leux*, 1575.[1]

The Protestants, it is said, considered the death of Henri at the hand of
Gabriel de Montgomery a judgement from God. Montgomery, a month
before the tourney accident, had been the officer sent by the king to arrest,
in open Session of Parliament, the Counsellor Anne du Bourg and other
secretly Calvinist magistrates. It is also to be remembered that by this
time the tournament ring was, in France, England and Italy, already
criticized as brutal and semi-barbarous; in Germany its vogue continued
much longer.

NOTE XI.   OTHER PORTRAITS OF FERNEL (p. 55)

OTHER printed portraits are:

1. In Sambucus' *Icones Veterum aliquot, ac recentium medicorum philo-
sophorumque*, Antwerp, 1574; 2°. It is no. 29 of the series. The shoulders
carry the same brocaded gown as in the woodcut of 1554. The profile is
turned left instead of right. On copper (?van d. Borcht). 2nd edition
1603.

2. A medallion woodcut likeness of Fernel is in the second edition
(valde aucta) of the '*Promptuarium Iconum*' of Guillaume Rouille, the

1 Pp. 128, 129; Henri Estienne said to be the author.

Lyons printer, p. 267; pars secunda, Lyons, 1577, and again 1581. The profile is turned to the left. The first edition (1553) does not contain Fernel. In all editions the series opens with a portrait of Adam, much as the fifteenth-century *De claris mulieribus* opened with a picture of Eve.

3. *Les Vrais Pourtraits et Vies des Hommes Illustres*, by André Thevet; 2°, Paris: Kerver's Widow and Chaudière; 1584, 2 vols. The portraits are of poets, scholars, etc. of antiquity, and a number of contemporaries of Thevet himself, among them Fernel; signed 'N. Larmessin sculpsit'. Each portrait occupies a folio page. Fernel's profile is to the right. It was copied, very poorly, for the Geneva edition of Fernel of 1679.

. 4. The *Imagines doctorum Vivorum e Variis Gentibus*, of Valerius Andreas, 1611 (Antwerp: D. Martinus), has a medallion engraving of Fernel; face in profile; the upper part of a human skeleton in the background. It is signed 'N. Larmessin sculp.' It was reproduced, reduced, in *Æsculape* for April, 1923, Paris.

5. The *Musaeum Historicum et Physicum*, of Johannes Imperialis (Venice, by the Giunta, 4°; 1640), contains in its first part, among fifty-two portraits, Fernel, along with Bembo, Scaliger, Aldrovandus, Lipsius, Critonius (i.e. Admirable Crichton), etc. The second part supplies notices of their work.

6. The *Pathologia* of 1638 (12°)—which may be regarded as Guy Patin's issue—has a medallion portrait, said to be 'new'. I have not seen the edition.

7. The Utrecht edition, edited by Joh. and O. Heurnius, 1656, has a frontispiece on copper, representing Fernel and the two editors seated at a table, Fernel between the Heurnes in earlier costume than they, and wearing the doctor's hat, whereas they are bare-headed. The scene is in the court of a hospital modified from Leyden, 1644.

8. An engraved portrait of Fernel, by P. Pinchard, is given in the Geneva folio edition of 1679. The likeness is hardly recognizable, and the engraving is poor; it is 'after' the portrait given by Thevet (*v. supra*). The printing of the volume, as Goulin remarked, is poor. Some copies are dated 1680.

Guy Patin (*Lettres*: letter 217; II, p. 59, edition 1692), writing to Falconet, 2 December, 1650, and again in a letter to Spon six years later, 6 March, 1656, mentions among pictures hanging in the room where he held his banquet for members of the Faculty, a portrait of Fernel. Goulin, writing in 1775 in Paris, says: 'In the chapel, where his epitaph is, there is a portrait of Fernel'; i.e. in the Church of St Jacques de la Boucherie. Goulin continues: 'the Paris Faculty has a portrait of him painted on canvas'. It may be that this is the portrait alluded to by Patin.

P. A. Capitaine, in his Paris thesis of 1925, says: 'As one enters the Salle des Pas-Perdus of the Faculty, the first bust to the left is that of Fernel'. The medal bearing the head and bust of Fernel, 1794, Paris, figured in the frontispiece to this book, is signed on the obverse and reverse 'N. Gatteaux'.

De Beauvillé, quoted by Figard (p. 41), speaks of there being as many as sixteen portraits extant of Fernel, and adds that in the south rose-window of Beauvais cathedral a portrait is given of Fernel in personification of St Luke.

NOTE XII. GUY PATIN (p. 59)

GUY PATIN (1601–1672) lives in his letters. For a readable and discriminating account of Patin, see *Annals of Medical History* (vol. IV, nos. 2, 3 and 4) by the editor, Dr Francis R. Packard, republished later, with some additions, as a volume: *Guy Patin and the Medical Profession in Paris in the seventeenth century*. This contains bibliographical references. Guy Patin succeeded Riolan fils as Dean of the Paris Faculty. The *Lettres* were first published in 1686, that is to say a selection of them (196). The Bibliothèque National has a collection of them, and the Library of the Faculté de Médecine of Paris another; the latter library was founded by Guy Patin. Osler writes: 'There have been some fifteen editions.[1] They have never been critically edited; curious fatalities have followed the attempts of Friare and others, and Friare himself, after issuing one volume (Paris, 1907) of what promised to be a definitive edition, died, leaving the work unfinished.' It seems that a number of the letters remain still unpublished.

NOTE XIII. THE TEXT OF THE 'PHYSIOLOGY' OF 1554 (p. 61)

ALTERATIONS in the *De Naturali Parte Medicinae* of 1542 when re-edited as the 'Physiology' of 1554, i.e. first part of the *Medicina*, were:

The dedicatory letter to the prince is replaced by one addressed to him as king. The Preface is altered in places toward the end. Physiology is somewhat differently and more fully defined.

Bk. i, chapters 1 and 2, of general introductory nature, are largely rewritten, and parts of the original chap. 1 are carried over, rephrased, into the re-written chap. 2. In chap. 16 the first two sentences of 1542 are omitted. These contained a reinsistence on the importance of studying anatomy from the actual dissection instead of from books and merely verbal description.

Bk. ii. The Preface is shortened and partly rewritten; its title, 'On different types of discipline, or the twofold road to proof', is omitted. It had distinguished in analysis the *a posteriori* from the *a priori*, and had

1 *Bibliotheca Osleriana*, p. 473.

cited, in illustration, Euclid's founding of geometry and arithmetic,
Ptolemy's founding of astronomy, and 'at last the founding of physiology
by Aristotle'.

Bk. v. 'On the Life-faculties.' Chap. 4 is largely rewritten; the final
sentence is recast. The marginal 'do plants distinguish between useful and
useless materials for nutriment' is omitted. Chap. 5 is an addition. It deals
with faculties of nutrition and secretion. It rejects the teaching of Plato
that plants feel pleasure and seek nutriment to draw enjoyment from it.
It elaborates the argument that they select food without *knowledge* of what
is useful. The 1542 chaps. 5–18 then follow, renumbered 6–19.

NOTE XIV. BOERHAAVE'S RECOMMENDATION OF BOOKS FOR MEDICAL CURRICULUM (p. 103)

IN the library of the Royal College of Surgeons, London, is a small MS.
volume of the early eighteenth century containing a list, alphabetically
arranged according to subject, of books recommended by Boerhaave to
his students for the doctorate in medicine, Leyden. It is written in latin,
presumably by some one attending Boerhaave's courses at that time. The
works recommended number in all 133. Appended to many of them is a
brief remark of characterization. Newton's *Principia* is 'indispensable'.
Boyle's works are recommended especially. Under 'pathologia' the work
recommended is Fernel's *Pathologia*. On Fernel's *Physiologia* the remark
is that nothing prior to Harvey is any longer of use. Nothing of Paracelsus comes into the list anywhere.

In 1667 Guy Patin praises a book which he has read in MS.; it should
find a publisher, because the best since the 'Pathology' of Fernel. Letter
482, p. 279, vol. III.

NOTE XV. NICOLAS LEONICENUS (p. 67)

NICOLAS LEONICENUS (1428–1524), physician and humanist, was a
translator of the *Aphorisms* into latin. He is the only contemporary whom
Fernel mentions by name in the *Dialogue* (ii, c. 7) or *Medicina*; Leonicenus
had then been dead 16 years. Fernel mentions him in dissent from him.
He is said to have suffered from epilepsy until the age of thirty, but he
lived to the age of ninety-six in the enjoyment of all his faculties. Asked
how to live in order to live long, his answer was 'Be frugal and merry'.

He corrected the corrupt text of Pliny's *Natural History*, and declared
Pliny mistaken in certain matters, and thus is said to have been the earliest
to bring to the mind of the time that the ancients were fallible.

Leonicenus was an enthusiast in medical astrology. A scholar himself,
he had among his friends Politian, Linacre, Augurello, Erasmus and
Scaliger. In a letter written to Erasmus, at the time of Leonicenus' death

(the same year as Linacre's), and preserved by him, *Epistolae Erasmi*, bk. 20 (Astruc, II, p. 18), the phrase ran: 'Leonicenus, the physician, a man born for eternity and to be reckoned among the last of the heroes and a relict of the age of gold.'

NOTE XVI. THOMAS LINACRE (p. 67)

THOMAS LINACRE (?1460–1524) is too well known to need general notice here. A physician to Henry VIII, he had been called to Court by Henry VII to be tutor to Prince Arthur. He founded the Royal College of Physicians of London (1518). He was an eminent medical humanist, and an early 'grecian'. Among those whom he instructed in greek were Sir Thomas More and Erasmus. His latin translations of Galen were highly valued and his latin grammar had international currency. The late Dr F. J. Payne suggested that Robert Browning's somewhat macabre verses, 'The Grammarian's Funeral', had Linacre in mind. Osler, in *Bibliotheca Osleriana*, adopted a similar view. In support of it Dr Archibald Malloch has recently brought forward evidence which seems more convincing (A. Malloch, 'Browning's copy of Linacre's latin grammar', *Proc. of the Charaka Club*, vol. VIII, New York, 1935). Browning was probably not at pains to depict the actual Linacre, any more than he was to present the actual Paracelsus. He used in each case the name to cover a lay-figure of his own fancy. The grim recluse pictured in the verses can hardly set forth the true Linacre, a courtier and a man of the world, as well as a persuasive leader of professional reform.

NOTE XVII. PASSAGE IN THE *PATHOLOGIA* OF 1567 (p. 102)

THE following passage is sometimes spoken of as an early record of a case of appendicitis with autopsy. I have submitted it to Professor H. R. Dean, Master of Trinity Hall, Professor of Pathology in the University; he kindly allows me to quote from his reply. 'The great violence of the pains, the abdominal distension and the faecal vomit all sound like a classical case of acute intestinal obstruction.' The passage translated, runs:

Similar to obstruction is constriction and narrowing of the intestine. This may be produced by the action of things ingested, whether foods, as bad bryony or astringent drenches, also by tumour of the mesentery or by the viscera pressing on the intestines and this is extremely common. It also happens from enterocele when the intestine comes down into the scrotum and is constricted by it as by a loop. Each of these ought to be perceptible of itself, and not indirectly.

It will not be irrelevant to insert at this point a notable example. A seven-year old girl was attacked by diarrhoea. For several days she passed, painlessly, a whitish evil-smelling oily matter. Her grandmother, anxious about the persistence of this discharge, took steps with other women to check it. By free doses of quince the bowel was so checked that that day and the following night nothing at all was passed. But the most agonizing pains and torments of the belly set in. The abdomen swelled up so much that it was thought that dropsy had suddenly come on. A doctor was summoned who suspected what was wrong. By repeatedly injecting clysters, at first mild, then more severe, he tried to bring away the noxious matter sticking to the bowel, and to reduce the pains by fomentation; but all in vain. Indeed, the dreadful pains increased, with frequent fainting fits, and finally with the vomiting of liquid faecal matter she passed miserably away. When the body was opened, the narrowed and constricted caecum was so impeded by the quince, blocking and stopping up its passage, that nothing could possibly get through that way. In result the bitter corrupt matter, being prevented from passing and barred, over-flowed and opened for itself an abnormal road into the abdominal cavity; the intestine was eaten through and perforated a little above the obstructed place, and by thus gaining an outlet or channel the matter had escaped and filled the entire capacity of the abdomen. Hence the extremely violent pains, the distension, the faintings, and, with the supervention of the foul vomiting, the swiftly following most cruel death. This case will be of value to those who too hastily stop or check an excessive and dangerous humour, whatever may be its source, to the very great disadvantage of their patients.

See *Univ. Med.* 1567, p. 303, i.e. *Pathologia*, lib. vi, cap. 11. Not in the earlier editions nor in the Rutilius Borgominierus of 1565, Ven. nor in the French transl. of the *Pathologia* by A.D.M. 1650.

NOTE XVIII. LAURENT JOUBERT'S PARADOXES (p. 108)

THIS is a small 8° volume published in 1566 (Lyons, at the Salamander, *in Via Mercuriali*). It contains two 'decads' of essays, the series numbering in fact only nine, much as with the prospectus of the *Erreurs Populaires*, which was never fulfilled. The first series had been published, without the author's permission (Lyons (Penot), 1561). The privilege is 'granted at Montpellier, December 1564'. The author, on the title, is described as of Dauphiné (Delphinas) and Professor of the Art of Medicine at Montpellier.

The two essays translated from their latin into french by Joubert fils, are (1) the last one of the second 'decad': 'that poisons on certain days cannot be given, and at certain times do not kill', and (2) the second one of the first 'decad': 'that in truth there are some people who can live several days and years without food'. These translations were supervised by Joubert père, and given a few short amplifications marked in brackets as being written by him. They are found appended to a Paris 8° edition (Claude Micard, 1587) of the *Erreurs Populaires*, but they must have appeared at least as early as 1580.

NOTE XIX. FRACASTOR ON CAUSE OF
SYPHILIS (p. 130)

'AND when you consider...you are bound to decide after deliberation that
the source and seat of the evil must exist in the air itself': ll. 119–21, bk. 1.

'Deeply he (Jupiter) pitied the miseries of the wretched Earth;...he
pitied it the strange contagion of a new disease; a disease no power of
human aid could assuage. The rest of the Gods assented;...and strange
rains fell from the troubled sky. Gradually the regions of heaven and the
wide voids of space received the pestilence; and the unknown taint made
its way through the empty air carrying contagion. Either when so many
stars came into conjunction with the blazing sun the fiery energy drew
many vapours from sea and land; and these mingled with thin air and
seized by the new taint conveyed a corruption too fine to be seen. Or
something other sent down from the upper air infected far and wide the
borders of the sky': ll. 238–55, bk. 1.

Fracastor. H. Wynne-Finch's translation, 1935.

That was Verona. What of Spain, where the disease first entered
Europe? De Oviedo's *Natural History of the Indies* (1525) tells how the
author, when a page at Court, had witnessed the outbreak of the strange
sickness on the return of Columbus' men from the Indies, and how later
he saw the disease in the Indies. It was commonly severe in Europeans
but mild in the Indians themselves. 'The natives were largely immune,
the Spaniards were not' is the comment of Mr Johnston Abraham
(Vicary Lecture, *Brit. J. of Surgery*, 1945, p. 229). Again a missionary,
de las Casas, in Hispaniola, records it was common knowledge that the
disease was there before Christianity. Again, the physician Ruy de Isla
of Barcelona states that it appeared there first with the return of
Columbus' sailors from the first voyage. The whole story hangs together.
Nevertheless, there was puzzlement for the earnest physician. A cloud
of witnesses attesting differently. Worst of all, the quacks—egregiously
among them Bombastus, soidisant paracelsus, inviting castigation as a
means to notoriety.

List of editions of the writings of
JEAN FERNEL

1A. *Monalosphaerium* 1527. 2B. *Cosmotheoria* 1528 (March). 3C. *De Proportionibus Liber* 1528 (November). 4–7D. *De Naturali Parte Medicinae* 1542. 8–16E. *De Vacuandi Ratione* 1545. 17–47F. *De Abditis Rerum Causis* [*Dialogi*] 1548. 48–54G. *Medicina* 1554. 55, 56H. *Opera Medicinalia* 1565. 57–88J. *Universa Medicina* 1567. 89–93K. *Therapeutices universalis* 1571. 94L. *Touching the outward Affects of the Body* [W. Clowes] 1575. 95–97M. *Febrium Curandarum Methodus Generalis* 1577. 98–101N. *De Luis Venereae perfectissima Cura Liber* 1579. 102–104P. *La Chirurgie* 1579. 105, 106Q. *Consilium pro epileptico* 1580. 107–121R. *Consiliorum Medicinalium Liber* 1582. 122S. *De Morbo Articulari* 1592. 123T. *Medici Antiqui* 1594. 124U. *Pharmacia* 1605. 125–127W. *Two Treatises on Eyesight* 1616. 128–133X. *Pathologia* 1638. 134Y. *De Morbis Universalibus et Particularibus* 1645. 135Z. *De Febribus, pathologiae Liber quartus* 1664. Ghosts.

(The bibliography by Goulin (*Mémoires*, 1775) contains eighty-seven items. Since then there has been only one further edition of a work by Fernel, namely the reissue (1879) by Le Pileur of the *De Luis Venereae Curatione*. Certain editions of Fernel were, however, not known to Goulin and have been added here.)

Locations of copies

AU, Aberdeen University; Bd, Bodleian; BM, British Museum; BN, Bibliothèque Nationale, Paris; CPL, College of Physicians, London; CSL, College of Surgeons, London; CSS, self; CUL, Cambridge University Library; EU, Edinburgh University; F, Dr J. F. Fulton; GCC, Gonville and Caius College, Cambridge; HC, Harvey Cushing Library, Yale; HMS, Dr H. M. Sinclair; MFP, Faculté de Médecine, Paris; MLM, Medical Library, Manchester; MSL, Medical Society of London; RPEd, Royal College of Physicians, Edinburgh; RS, The Royal Society; RSM, Royal Society of Medicine, London; SG, Surgeon-General's Library, Washington; TCD, Trinity College, Dublin; TrC, Trinity College, Cambridge; UG, University of Glasgow; Vat., Vatican Library. [Omission of a location indicates no copy at that location. A numeral signifies no. of copies, e.g. EU² indicates 2 copies.]

A. *Monalosphaerium* 1527 (N.S.)

1.A. Joannis Fer-| nelii Ambianatis Mo-| nalosphaerium, partibus constans | quatuor. | Prima, generalis horarij & structu-| ram, & usum, in exquisitam mona-| losphaerij Cognitionem praemittit. | Secūda, mobilium solemnitatum, | criticorumq dierū rationes, mul- | ta brevitate complectitur. | Tertia, quascūq ex motu primi mo- | bilis deprōptas utilitates elargitur. | Quarta, geometrica praxin brevius-culis demōstrationibus dilucidat. | Haec sanè cūcta excutit mona- | losphaerium: quorū capita sub- | sequentes facies ostentant. | *Parisiis.* In aedibus *Simonis Colinaei.* 1526. 2°. 6ff. unnumbered + 36ff. numbered recto only. Sign. a–g by 6; roman letters. Woodcut initials on stippled ground: marginal notes. BM, AU, BN, Bd, CUL, EU², F, MSL, RS, HC, TrC, HMS. Two variants of the title-page, both with the same decorative border (assigned by Mr E. P. Goldschmidt to Oronce Finé (d .1555), the mathematician), *v.s.* fig. 2, p. 13, for the scientific folios de Colines was publishing and first used for the 'Arithmetic' of Jean Martin Siliceus in this same year. One variant says 1526, the other 1527. The decorated border consists of an interlaced ribbon knotwork, in white on a criblé black ground, carrying figures of (to left) Astronomy, Music, Geometry and Arithmetic and (to right) Ptolemy, Orpheus, Euclid and Algus; at top the arms of France, at bottom of Dauphiné (Oronce Finé was of Dauphiné). Text with woodcuts. Colophon: 'Excudebat Simon Colinaeus Anno Vir-ginei Partus M.D.XXVII. Nonis Martii.' Dedication: 'Apud celebratissimum divae Barbarae gymnasium, ad calendas Februarias, 1526', to Jacques de Govea, 'numeris omnibus absolutissimo Viro, ac sacrae theologiae doctori celeberrimo'.

Among preliminaries contains complimentary latin elegiacs to the author by a pupil, Denis Armenault, 'Senonensis', who likewise contributed lines to Fernel's next volume, the *Cosmotheoria.* On the verso of leaf 36 are twenty lines of latin elegiacs addressed to young fellow-pupils, one of them a Portuguese. The Goveas were of Portuguese extraction.

A volume, or album, of plates was issued accompanying the *Monalosphaerium* and was priced higher than the book itself (Ph. Renouard, *Simon de Colines,* p. 428).

B.   *Cosmotheoria*   1528 March (N.S.)

2.B.   Joannis Ferne | lii ambianatis cosmo | theoria libros duos complexa. | Prior, mūdi totius & formam & com | positionem: ejus subinde partium | ...situs et magnitudines: orbiū | tandem motus...re | serat. | Posterior, ex motibus, siderū loca & passiones disquirit: interspersis do | cumentis...additum | ad astronomicas tabulas supplēditā | tibus etc. Simon de Colines, Paris, 1527. 2°. 6ff. unnumbered + 46ff. numbered on recto. Sign. A–H by 6, I by 4, the f. I, iiii signed by mistake I, ii. BM, AU, BN, Bd, EU² (the two variant issues), F, MFP, RS, HC, Méd. Fac. Libr. Montpellier (Renouard). Text with woodcuts. Title-page with same decorated border as no. 1; two variants of the title-page as to date, one 1527, the other 1528. The colophon 'An- | no Christi, caelorum et siderum conditoris | M.D.XXVII ad Calendas | Februarii. |' in both is dated 1527. The dedicatory preface to John III of Portugal is dated by Fernel 'pridie nonas Februarias ex alma Parisiorum accademia, 1528'. On the assumption that this last is O.S. Goulin dates the book 1529; but that is incompatible with 1527 in the colophon of both issues. This book contains the measurement of a degree of meridian by Fernel and a description of how he carried it out. There are a fresh set of complimentary verses to the author by his pupil Denis Armenault of Sens.

C. *De Proportionibus Liber* 1528 (November)

3.C. 'Joannis Fer | nelii Ambianatis | de proportionibus Libri duo. | Prior, qui de simplici proportio- | ne est, & magnitudinum & nu- | merorum tum simplicium tum | fractorum rationes edocet. | Posterior, ipsas proportiones cō- | parat: earumq rationes colligit. | Parisiis | Ex aedibus Simonis Colinaei | 1528 |. 2°. 4ff. unnumbered + 24ff. numbered on recto only. Sign. A by 4, B–E by 6. Title-page decoration as in nos. 1 and 2. An album of plates was issued with this volume entitled 'Instrumenta mathematica Fernelii de proportionibus libris depicta, perbelle concinnata' and priced at 12 sols (see Ph. Renouard, p. 428). Woodcut initials. One woodcut figure in text. Marginals. BM, AU, BN, Bd, EU², F, MFP, HC, Tr.C.

D. *De Naturali Parte Medicinae* 1542

4.D1. Joannis Fernelij Ambianatis, | De naturali parte medicinae Libri septem, | ad Henricum Francisci Galliae | Regis filium. | Apud Simonem Colinaeum. | Parisiis. | Anno M.D.XLII. | Cum privilegio. | Simon de Colines: (at the Quatre Evangelistes), Paris, 1542. 2°. 10ff. + 168 (wrongly numbered 165) ff. UG, CSS. Renouard (p. 357) cites copies at Ajaccio, Bordeaux, Dijon, Valence, and Bibl. Ste-Geneviève, Paris; *v.s.* fig. 1, p. 3, fig. 3, p. 21, fig. 12, p. 61.

Mentioned in Conr. Gesner's *Bibliotheca Universalis*, 1545; Goulin, Paris, 1775, could not find a copy: 'je conclus...fort rare.' Renaudin, *Biograph. Universelle*, Paris, 1857, vol. XIV: 'édition extrêmement rare'. Only two copies seem known outside France. Guy Patin, writing to Falconet, 27 December 1658, says erroneously of this book: 'Sa' (i.e. Fernel's) 'Physiologie ne fut imprimée que trois ans après, scavoir l'an 1538': *Lettres*, edit. Paris, 1692, II, p. 131, lett. 248.

The copy (31 cm. + 21 cm.) in the Hunterian Library, Glasgow University, leather-boards, has the arms of the dauphin blind-stamped, and the fleur-de-lis gold-stamped. The large initials in the text are illuminated and coloured. The text is rubricated and enclosed by a red line hand-inserted. Perhaps this copy belonged to Henri II when dauphin, to whom as dauphin the work was dedicated; the Hunterian Library contains a volume from Diane de Poitier's library, with binding carrying the monogram combining Diane and Henry's initials.

5.D2. [Gryphius, Joh.: (nephew of S. Gryphius, Lyons)] Venetiis 1547. De Naturali | ... Septem. | Joanne Farnelio (*sic*) Ambianate autore: | Mendis quamplurimis, incuria praetermissis, | praesertim in dictionibus Graecis, expurga- | ti. Index insuper tertia plus fere par | te locupletior redditus. The Gryphius device on title with 'Virtute Duce | Comite Fortuna'. 26 unnumbered leaves (title, dedication, index, errata, two blanks) + 260 leaves numbered—italics throughout, except for the marginals, which are roman. 8°. Vat, F, SG, CSS. Among items added here to the index of the 1st edition is 'Dialogorum Ioan. Ferne. lib. i, 90a', a reference to one of the marginals indicating that Fernel's 'Dialogue' was already extant, though printed only in 1548, i.e. after this 2nd edition of the 'Physiology' had appeared; *v.s.* fig. 4, p. 21. The index is greatly enlarged. Printer's name is not given, but the Gryphius mark and motto are on the title-page; *v.s.* fig. 18, p. 104.

Jean Gryphe printed at Venice, 1541–57, and the press continued to 1585; his mark and motto are like those of the famous Lyons house; his productions rarely state *where* printed. Baudrier (*Bibliogr. Lyonnais*) suggests they encouraged a lucrative confusion with the Lyons house. The book here dealt with does state 'Venice'; perhaps expressly to show it was not infringing the French privilege of the Paris 1542 edition.

6.D3. Joan. Tornaesius et Guliel. Gazeius, Lyons, 1551. 16°. 8 pp. + index 40 pp. + text 655 pp. BN, Vat, MFP, UG, HMS, CSS. The index is as in the 1st edition and less full than in the 1547 edition.

7.D4. (In french.) Les VII Livres de la Physiologie, composez en Latin par Messire Jean Fernel,...Traduits en Francois par Charles de Saint Germain, Escuyer, Docteur en la Faculté de Médecine, Conseiller & Médecin ordinaire du Roy. Chez Jean Guignard le Jeune, etc. A Paris. 1655. 8°. pp. 11 + 773. F, MFP, HMS. Not given by Goulin.

Privilege granted to Widow Jean Le Bouc, for nine years, 28 April 1638, and by her accorded to Guignard père et fils. 'Achevé d'imprimer pour la premiere fois le 21 Sept. 1655.' This translation is not from the *De naturali parte Medicinae*, but from the *Medicina* (1554).

E.   *De Vacuandi Ratione*   1545

8.E1. De Vacuandi ratione liber. Christian Wechel at the Shield of Basle, rue St Jacques; and at the Pegasus, rue de Beauvais, Paris, 1545. 8°. 141 pp. BN, F, MFP, SG, UG. Christian Wechel printed for Erasmus and for Rabelais. De Colines, who had printed for Fernel, was already ill in 1546; he was also perhaps too expensive. Twenty-one chapters.

BIBLIOGRAPHICAL LIST OF FERNEL'S WORKS 191

9.E2. Joan. Tornaesius et Guliel. Gazeius, Lyons, 1548. 16°. BM, MFP, F. First de Tournes' issue of a Fernel edition; de Tournes had a Paris agent in 1561 (Pichon and Vicaire's *Documents*, etc., Paris, 1895). Baudrier states that Gazius first joined de Tournes in 1556, but this book and 6.D3 bring the date to 8 years earlier.

10.E3. Ex officina Erasmiana, Venice, 1548. 8°. CSS. Italics throughout.

11.E4. Vincent Valgrisius, Venice, 1549. 8°. BM, Vat, MFP, SG.

12.E5. Gulielm. Rouillius, Lyons, 1549. 12°. pp. 156 + 2. AU, BN, MFP, CSS. Retains original dedication. R. a generous benefactor to Lyons.

From 1554 onwards the *De Vacuandi Ratione* appeared incorporated in the *Medicina* and *Universa Medicina* as bk. ii of the 'Therapeutics'.

13.E6. Hanau, 1603. 8°. (Cited by Alb. Haller, *Stud. medicum*, p. 850.)

14.E7. Joann. Saurius, Frankfort, 1612. 12°. Included with *Schola Salernitana*. CSS.

15.E8. Joann. Saurius, Frankfort, 1631. 12°. Like no. 14. CSS.

16.E9. Jacob Stoer, Genevae, 1638. 16°. Printed following *Medicina Salernitana*, 'edited by Arnoldus Villanovanus'; an excerpt from *De Vacuandi Ratione*, c. 20, 'emissi observatio', and occupies pp. 402–5. CSS.

F. *De Abditis Rerum Causis,* referred to by Fernel as *Dialogi*

1548

17.F1. De abditis rerum causis libri ij, ad Henricum Franciae regem christianissimum, cum privilegio regis ad sexennium; apud Christianum Wechelum, Paris, 1548. Fernel from this date onwards is styled *Ambianus*, not *Ambianas*, e.g. also item No. 10. Plancy uses *Ambianus* in the *Vita*. J. Sylvius, likewise from the Amiens countryside, called himself *Ambianus*. AU, BN, F², MFP. 255 pp. + index + privilege in french. Title-page occurs in two forms, both carrying the Wechel Pegasus emblem. One form has 'sub scuto Basiliensi in vico Jacobaeo'; *v.s.* fig. 8, p. 35; the other 'Sub Pegaso in vico bellovacensis et é regione apud Carolum Perier'; *v.s.* fig. 7, p. 35. Charles Périer was a son of Jean Périer of the 'Jeu de Paume of St Jean de Latran', in the rue St Jean de Beauvais, by his first wife. Christian Wechel married Michelle Robillart in her widowhood, Jean Périer's second wife. He removed to the Jeu de Paume, changing its name to the Cheval-Volant (Pegasus). The Pegasus, the sign appearing in so many editions of Fernel, stood higher up than the College of Beauvais in the rue de St Jean de Beauvais, and on the opposite side of the street. H. Périer was still publishing in Paris in the seventeenth century Riolan's Commentary on Fernel.

18.F2.   Andreas Arrivabenus, Venice, 1550. 8°. pp. 24 + 310. BN, SG, CSS. 'At the house of Peter and John Maria de Nicolinis de Sabio, but at the expense of And. Arrivabenus at the sign of the Well.' The dedicatory letter by the publisher is to the Arrivabenus, 'eminent philosopher and physician'. Well printed on good paper.

19.F3.   Christian Wechel, Paris, 1551. 2°. Two forms of title-page; one with Pegasus device: Bd, MFP, TCD, CSS; the other, CSS, has for device a woodcut of a carved screen with four actor-masks carrying a central oval cameo on which Christ at the well and the woman of Samaria. Below the device, 'Pariiis [sic], Apud Jacobum Dupuys, via ad D. Joannem Lateranensem, è regione collegij Cameracensis, sub signo Samaritanae'. This device plays on the name Dupuys. Jacques du Puys had for his first wife Catherine, a daughter of Josse Badius. A brother, Mathurin, was also a printer, in the rue St Jacques, at the sign of 'L'homme Sauvage' and of 'Froben'. The rue St Jean de Latran ran, more or less parallel with the river, but some way from it, from the rue St Jean de Beauvais across to the rue St Jacques above the church of St Jean de Latran. On the verso of the title-page is the privilege, printed in italics. Then 7 ff. of index followed by four couplets in greek, in honour of Fernel, by Jacques Goupyl, physician. These issues call themselves 'second edition'. Figs. 24 and 25. Similar privilege as in 17.F1.

J. G. Goupyl succeeded (1548) J. Sylvius as medical professor at the Royal College (later Coll. de France), Paris. A humanist and collector of MSS., the destruction of his collection is said to have contributed to his death (1563). He was the teacher of T. Jordan, of Brunn. He listed the names of trees, fruits, birds, and fish in greek and latin with their French equivalents (Paris, 1545). He edited Aretaeus, Rufus of Ephesus, Paulus of Aegina, and others; some of them were printed by Turnebus his colleague and Regius Professor of Greek at the Royal College.

The Pegasus device occurs at the end-page irrespective of the two forms of title-page. Large and smaller picture-initials identical with those of the 1st edition, but a new picture initial at the beginning of the index.

Goulin knew a copy in St-Germain-des-Prés, but remarks that it must be a rare edition because the *only* mention of a copy is in the Bodleian Catalogue of 1674; doubtless the copy now there. Next year (1552) Christian Wechel died, and Plancy, Fernel's pupil, is found publishing his 'Plutarch' at Andreas Wechel's.

20.F4.   Andreas Wechel, Paris, 1560. 8°. pp. 426 + index. BN, CSL, MFP, F, CSS. Well printed on good paper.

21.F5.   Rutilius Borgominierus, Venice, 1565, with the *Medicina*; see no. 55.

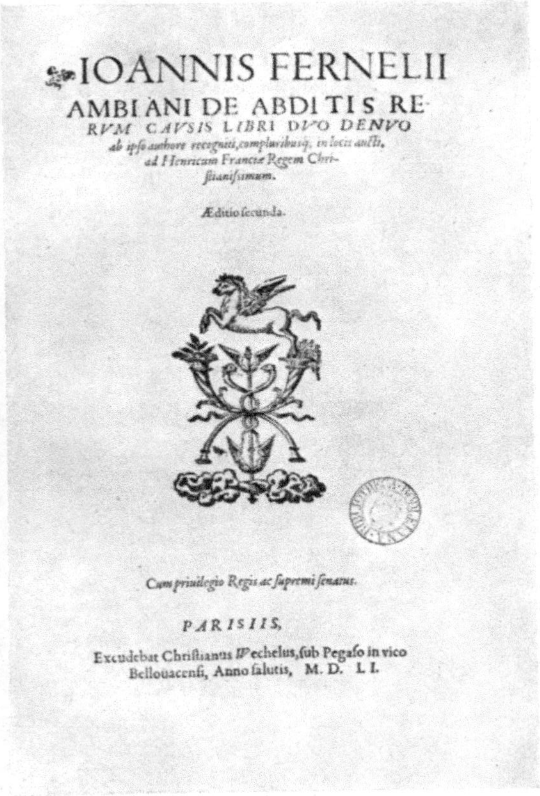

IOANNIS FERNELII
AMBIANI DE ABDITIS RE-
RVM CAVSIS LIBRI DVO DENVO
ab ipso authore recogniti, compluribusq; in locis aucti,
ad Henricum Franciæ Regem Chri-
stianissimum.

Æditio secunda.

Cum priuilegio Regis ac supremi senatus.

PARISIIS,

Excudebat Christianus Wechelus, sub Pegaso in vico
Bellouacensi, Anno salutis, M. D. L I.

IOANNIS FERNELII
AMBIANI DE ABDITIS RE-
RVM CAVSIS LIBRI DVO DENVO
ab ipso authore recogniti, compluribusq; in locis aucti,
ad Henricum Franciæ Regem Chri-
stianissimum.

Æditio secunda.

Cum priuilegio Regis ac supremi senatus.

PARISIIS,

Apud Iacobum Dupuys, via ad D. Ioannem Lateranensem, è
regione collegij Cameracensis, sub signo Samaritanæ.
Anno salutis, M. D. L I.

Fig. 24. (By courtesy of the Bodleian Library). Fig. 25.

Figs. 24, 25. Variant title-pages of the 2nd edition of the 'Dialogue', 2°, Paris, 1551.

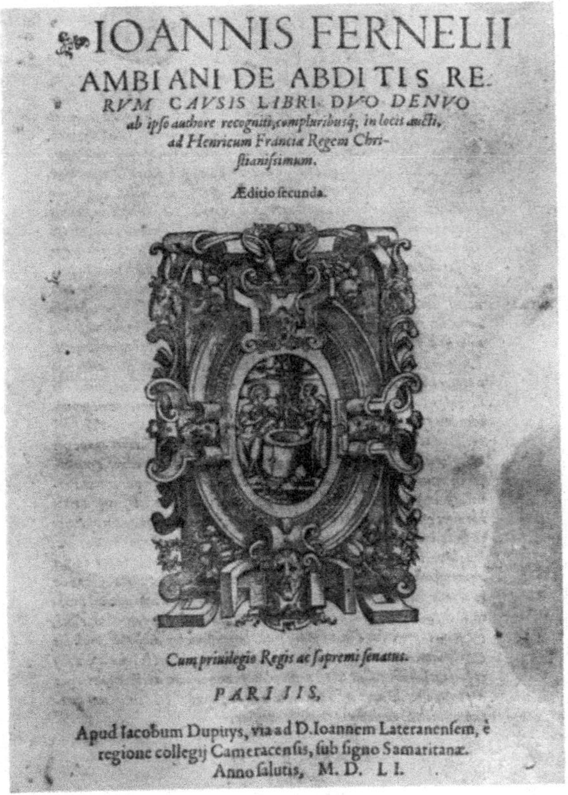

22.F6. Jordan Ziletti, Venice, 1566–7. 2°. 2 vols. Collection, called 'Venet. 2da', of syphilis tracts, containing extract from the 'Dialogue', bk. ii, c. 14, in vol. I, pp. 524 and 527; by Luvigini (Aloysius Luisinus): 'De Morbo Gallico omnia quae extant apud omnes Medicos Cuiuscunque nationis'.

The special tract by Fernel devoted to *lues venerea* had not appeared, owing to Fernel's death, when this collection was made. Aloisio Luvigini was a physician of Udine and Venice. BM, AU, Vat, Bd, CSL, F, CSS, etc.

23.F7. Andreas Wechel, Paris, 1567. 2°, with *Universa Medicina*; see no. 57.

24.F8. Andreas Wechel, Frankfort, 1574. 8°. Wechel left Paris, because of religion, in 1573. The same Pegasus device as in Paris. The 'Dialogue' is in vol. II of the *Universa Medicina*, no. 59.

25.F9. Andreas Wechel, Frankfort, 1575. 8°. pp. 272 + index. AU, BN, UG. Part of no. 60.

26.F10. Andreas Wechel, Frankfort, 1577. 2°. Part of no. 61.

27.F11. Andreas Wechel, Frankfort, 1578. Part of no. 62.

28.F12. Andreas Wechel, Frankfort, 1581. 8°. Title + aa6 + (13–272). AU, Vat, F, MFP, MSL, SG, GCL, CSS. Andreas Wechel died in November this year. Uniform with no. 68 printed in the same year.

29.F13. Heirs of Andreas Wechel, Frankfort, 1592. 2°. Bd. MLM. Part of no. 70.

30.F14. Heirs of Andreas Wechel. C. Marnius and J. Aubrius, Frankfort, 1593. 8°. AU, UG, F. Part of no. 71.

31.F15. Thomas Soubron and Moyses des Prez, Lyons, 1597. 8°. SG. Uniform with no 72.

32.F16. Baretius et Socii, Venice, 1599. 2°. Extract as in no. 22, given in the *Aphrodisiacus sive de Lue Venerea*, of Luvigini, I, pp. 527–8. BM, EU, etc.

33.F17. Thomas Soubron and Jean Veyrat, Lyons, 1602. 2°. SG. Part of no. 73.

34.F18. Thomas Soubron and Jean Veyrat, Lyons, 1604. 8°. F, SG.

35.F19. Petrus de la Rovière, Orleans, 1604. 8°. Pp. 264 + index. F (2 issues). CSS. Part of no. 74.

36.F20. B. Vincent, Lyons, 1605. 8°. BN, SG, pp. 264.

37.F21. C. Marny and heirs. J. Aubry, Frankfort, 1607. 8°. AU, Bd, MFP, SG. Part of no. 76.

38.F22. Again 1608. F.

39.F23. C. Marny, Hanau (Hanoviae), 1610. 2°. Bd, CUL², MSL, F. TrC. Part of no. 77.

40.F24. Claude Morillon, Lyons, 1615. 2°. Part of no. 78.

41.F25. Geneva, 1627. 8°. MFP, SG.

42.F26. Peter Chouet, Geneva, 1638. 8°. Vat, BN, Bd, MFP, SG, CSS. Part of no. 82, with separate pagination but signatures continuous.

43.F27. Like no. 42, but 1644. MFP, SG, CSS.

44.F28. Francis Hacke, Leyden, 1644. 8°. AU, CSL, CUL, MSL, F, HMS, GC, TrC. The 'Dialogue' is paragraphed per speaker for first time. Part of no. 85.

45.F29. Typis Gisberti a Zyll and Theod. ab Ackersdijck, Utrecht, 1656. 4°, with no. 83. BM, AU, BN, RPEd, CUL², MFP, F, MSL, CSS, HMS (several variants). The 'Dialogue' is paragraphed per speaker. Part of no. 86.

46.F30. John A. Langerak and John and Herm. Verbeck, Leyden, 1728. 2°. Extract as in no. 22, Luvigini's *Aphrodisiacus*, now reprinted at request of Herm. Boerhaave, but still without Fernel's special tract (N). BM, CSL, RSM, Vat, AU, SG, F.

47.F31. G. Masson, Paris, 1879. 8°. Extract bk. ii, c. 4, and in french, by Le Pileur; see below, no. 101.

G. *Medicina* 1554

48.G1. Medicina. Andreas Wechel, Paris, 1554. 2°. BN², CSL, F (the Riolan-Wignerot copy), MFP, RSM, SG, UG², HMS, CSS. Contains *Physiologiae*, lib. VII; *Pathologiae*, lib. VII; *Therapeutice*, lib. III; the woodcut portrait (profile to right) for the first time. The *Physiologia* says it has been revised and amplified from the *De naturali parte Medicine* (cap. 4, lib. v is mostly new). Dedicatory letter to King Henri II. Two copies in the Bibliothèque Nationale, one said to be King Henri's copy. Under Fernel's portrait a couplet in greek by Gul. Plancy, whose Doctorate of Medicine (Paris) dates this year. CSS copy, 37 cm. × 24 cm.; gilt-tooled on all three edges; the pages lineated, i.e. contained by red hand-ruled lines. The index of the *Physiologia* is not so full as in the 1542 edition, and still less so than in the 1547 edition. *V.s.* figs. 10, p. 54; 16, p. 92; 17, p. 100.

The 'appendicitis' case is not contained in this edition (my notice was first called to this by Dr J. F. Fulton). The second book of the 'Therapeutics' is the *De Vacuandi Ratione*, slightly rewritten and divided into 20 chapters instead of 21. The *Pathologia* appears for the first time. (*Christian* Wechel had not ceased to print; he continued in business till 1563; Ph. Renouard.)

49.G2. Balthassar Constantinus, Venice, 1555. 8°. In three parts, ff. 238 + 20, 219 + 26, 80 (misprinted '70') + 11. Vat, F, RSM, SG, RPEd.

50.G3. Peter Boselli, Venice, 1555. 8° (small). In three parts. CUL², GCC. The *Pathologia* part only: F, CSS. The title-page preceding the *Physiologia* is common to all three parts. Printer's device, a legionary with drawn sword mounted on a bull galloping, contained in a decorative border with angel, putti, a mask and fruits. Vertically to either side 'A furore rusticorum libera nos, Domine'. Woodcut historiated capitals. *V.s.* fig. 19, p. 104.

51.G4. Caesar Farina, Lyons; printer J. Ausult, 1564. 8°. 87+57+33 pp. BN, Bd, F, MFP, SG, CSS. pp. 757. F. moved to Turin, 1570.

52.G5. Jordan Ziletti, Venice, 1566–7. 2°. 2 vols. Collection, called 'Venet. 2da', of syphilis tracts, containing extracts from the *Pathologia*, on syphilis (bk. vi, c. 20); collection by Aloisio Luvigini, *v. supra*, no. 22.

53.G6. John A. Langerak, and John and Bernard Verbeck, Leyden, 1728. 2°. Reprint of Luvigini, containing extract as in no. 52 above.

54.G7. G. Masson, Paris, 1879. 8°. Same extract, given also in french, by Le Pileur. Cf. above.

H.   *Opera Medicinalia*   1565

55.H1. Opera Medicinalia. Rutilius Borgominierus, Venice, 1565. 4°. Pp. 56 + 13 + 569 (misprinted 565). F, SG, CSS. The *Medicina* with the *De Abditis Rerum Causis*. Goulin gives the date of this as 1564.

56.H2. Francis de Portunaris, Venice, 1566. 4°. Vat, SG, HMS, CSS. Closely similar to the next preceding, except for the title-page.

J.   *Universa Medicina*   1567

57.J1. Universa Medicina: physiologia, vii, pathologia, vii, therapeutice vii, De abditis rerum causis ii. Gulielmi Plantii elimata. Andreas Wechel, Paris, 1567. 2°. AU, CUL, F, MFP, HMS, RSM, EU, CSS.

The *De Abditis Rerum Causis* had been intended originally to come next after the 'Physiology', as the repetition word shows. The edition has the introductory letter of Plancy, March 1567, Paris. The printing of the text was finished 27 February 1567. The profile woodcut of Fernel of the 1554 *Medicina* is reproduced. There are 2 pages of laudatory verses in latin by Simon Poncetius of Melun, D.M., and by René Gervais, Fran. Thorius Bellio and Esaius Febius; in greek by Bellio and André Ribaudel; and the greek couplet by Plancy under the woodcut portrait. This volume contains for the first time, at p. 303, the 'appendicitis' case (bk. vi, c. 9).

58.J2. J. Arbillius. 1569. 8°. CUL (part only), SG.

59.J3. Andreas Wechel, Frankfort, 1574. 8°. 2 vols. BN. Andreas Wechel had left Paris for Frankfort, and this was one of the earliest of his books there. This is the first edition to contain the letter by Crato of Craftheim. Goulin points out that after removal to Germany the poor quality of the paper there impaired Wechel's printing.

60.J4. Similar to no. 59, but dated 1575. BN. Vol. I contains the *Physiologia* and the *Pathologia*, and the index; vol. II contains the *Therapeutices*, and the 'Dialogue'.

61.J5. Andreas Wechel, Frankfort. 1577. 2°. SG, EU. 2 pp. letter to Andrew Wechel from John Crato of Craftheim, physician-in-chief to the emperor, dated from Vienna, May 1574. Like no. 59, but after the 'Therapeutics', comes the 'General Treatment of Fevers', 'nunquam antea editus', without Lamy's letter. Contains the 'Dialogue', separately.

The work on fevers is doubtless that mentioned by Plancy in his Preface of 1567 as being left 'completed' by Fernel. Plancy had evidently meant to issue it at no remote date, for he concludes his letter to the reader with 'Interim, vale'. Cf. also *Appendix, Vita*, p. 164.

62.J6. Andreas Wechel, Frankfort, 1578. 2°. CSS. Like no. 61, except for date on title-page.

63.J7. A. Marsilius, Lyons, 1578. 2°. SG. M. italian from Lucca.

64.J8. ? Paris, 1578. MFP.

65.J9. Jacob Stoer (Genuae), 1578. 2°. Prelim. + 657 pp. + index. BN. Contents like no. 57, with addition of the 'Treatment of Fevers' and of the 'Perfect Cure of Syphilis'. The latter seems only to occur in copies issued in 1580, and Goulin states the *Curatio* carried the printed date, 1580. Goulin had seen a copy of this edition in which a former owner had written that a MS. of the *Cura. perf.*, which Lamy had, did not contain the three formulae found at the conclusion of this printed version.

66.J10. Basle, 1579. 8°. BN.

67.J11. Jacob Stoer, Genuae, 1580. 2°. BN. Contains along with *Meth. febrium curand. general.* the tract on syphilis, paged together (63 pp.) under the title *Febrium ac luis Venereae curatio methodica libris duobus comprehensa*; J. Lamy, editor. Portrait.

68.J12. Andreas Wechel, Frankfort, 1581. 8° (small). F, HMS, CSS. Calls itself 4th ed., 3 vols. Has the *De Luis Venereae Curatione* and the *Meth. febrium curand. general.* with Lamy's letter in vol. 2. The woodcut of 1554 has been recut; the greek type is fresh. A. Wechel died this year. From this (1581) Wechel edition Le Pileur issued his text (and translation) of the *De Luis Venereae Curatione*, etc. in Paris, 1879. (CSS copy is in blind-stamped pigskin, dated 1590, and carrying the arms and crest of 'Augustus Herczog zu Sachssen und Churfurst'. Edges tooled with loop-pattern.) Andr. Wechel died, Nov. 1, of this year.

69.J13. Junta and Pa. Guittius, Lyons, 1586. 2°. BM, AU. Contains also *Febrium* and *De Luis Venereae Curatione*. On the death of Jeanne Giunta (1585) her son-in-law, J. B. Regnaud, who managed her business, added to the imprint the name of the head-workman, Paolo Guittio. The plan was discontinued in 1587. The Junta were printing also in Venice and Florence.

70.J14. Heirs of Andreas Wechel; G. Marny and J. Aubry, Frankfort, 1592. 2°. Vat, Bd, CPL, MLM, GCC. Contains the *Meth. febrium curand. general.* with Lamy's letter and the *De Luis Venereae Curatione*. Grüner's reprint of this latter is from this edition. Grüner (cf. no. 99) seemingly did not know of the 4th edition (1581).

71.J15. As no. 70, 1593. 8°. CSL, RSM.

72.J16. Thomas Soubron and Moyses des Prez, Lyons, 1597. 8°. 2 vols. SG. Calls itself 6th edition (J. Riolan père's *Compendium Universae Medicinae* appeared the year following (1598) this edition, in Paris, H. Perier. 8°.) In vol. 1 some prescriptions by Tagault, Sylvius and de Flexelle—Fernel's old enemy—are given. Vol. 11 includes the 'Fevers' and the 'Cure of Lues venerea'.

73.J17. Jean Veyrat and Thomas Soubron, Lyons, 1601–2. 2°. 2 vols. Vat. BN, MFP, SG. Calls itself 7th edition. Preface by Plancy (of 1567) omitted. The *Conciliorum* has the second letter from Capell to Le Paulmier.

74.J18. P. de la Rovière, Orleans, 1604. 8°. Vat, BN, F, MFP, HMS, CSS. Two issues of this, one sometimes said to contain Plancy's *Vita* (if so, first issue of the *Vita*). My copy has not the *Vita*.

75.J19. J. de Gabiano and S. Girardi, Lyons, 1605. 8°. 2 vols. HMS. The second volume only was seen by Goulin. Goulin remarks of the edition 'that it can disappear without exciting the least regret'.

76.J20. Claude Marny and heirs of Jean Aubry, Frankfort, 1607. 8°. 2 vols. AU, BN, Bd, MFP, SG. Calls itself 6th edition, to which is added Fernel's *Vita* (by Plancy). The MS. used for the *Vita* (first publication) was not in Plancy's autograph but was a copy in another hand. '6th edition' may mean the 6th octavo edition, but five previous 8° editions by this firm are not known. If issues of 2° size as well as 8° are included, this is the eighth by this firm. Vol. 1 contains the *Vita*, the appreciations by de Thou and by Ste Marthe (for the first time). The second volume bears Hanoviae (i.e. Hanau) instead of Francofurti.

77.J21. Claude Marny, heir of John and Andrew Marny and partners, Hanoviae (Hanau), 1610. 2°. BN, Bd, RPEd, CSL, CUL², F, MFP,

MLM, MSL, TrC, EU, UG. This edition styles itself '6th', perhaps as being the 6th folio edition. The *Vita* is without marginals, except one which runs, 'LII forse scripsit ita enim aevi clariss. nostri historici et chronologi'. The historian referred to is de Thou, in bk 21 of his *History of His Own Time*, there giving the age of Fernel as fifty-two. This is the issue for the last time of a work of Fernel's from the firm of Wechel and his successors. Includes the 'Fevers' and the 'Cure of Lues venerea', the latter without the letter from Gisellinus.

78.J22. Claude Morillon, Lyons, 1615. 2°. EU, HMS. Calls itself 8th edition. Excellent print and paper. Does not contain the *Vita*. M. styles himself printer to the Duchess de Montpensier.

79.J23. Stephen Gamonetus, Geneva, at Peter and Jacob Chouet's, 1619. 4°. 1172 pp. of text. MFP, EU, HMS. 'Jamais au nombre des belles productions typographiques': Goulin.

80.J24. Geneva, 1627. 8°. BN, Bd, MFP.

81.J25. *Typis Jacobi Stoer*, Geneva, 1637. 4°. F, MFP, SG, EU, CSS. Title red and black, in figurated border; pp. 1172 + indices, etc. Additional consilia by Joh. Capellan, Sim. Petreius, cf. p. 38, one mentioning Flexelle (q.v.). Does not contain *Vita*. The 'Dialogue' is not paragraphed.

82.J26. Peter Chouet, Geneva, 1638. 8°. Vat, BN, Bd, MFP, SG, HMS, TrC, CSS. In Trinity College, Cambridge, a copy which states 'apud J. Crispin'.

83.J27. Geneva, 1643. 8°. MFP, RS.

84.J28. Jacob Chouet, Geneva, 1644. 8°. MFP, SG, CSS.

85.J29. Francis Hacke, Leyden, 1644-5. 8°. 2 vols. BM, BN, RPEd, CSL, HMS, CUL², F, MFP, MSL, TrC, UG. Notes, etc., by someone who 'wished to remain anonymous'; Goulin says it became known that 'it was Heurnius'. Vol. 1 has a frontispiece engraving, showing Fernel upright at a table, in a building containing dead and sick, and two figures seated listening to him. Hacke was leader of the 26 Leyden publishers then.

The *Vita* has marginals including 'Reginam curavit', a mistake for Diane de Poitiers. The 'Dialogue' is called 'de abditarum rerum causis', (not in all issues). It is paragraphed per speaker for the first time. The individual works are given in a fresh order of arrangement.

86.J30. Gisbert à Zijll and Theodor ab Ackersdijck, Utrecht, 1656. 4°. BM, AU, BN, RPEd, CUL², MFP, MSL, HMS⁴, CSS. Describes itself as augmented by John and his son, Otho Heurnes, of the Leyden Academy. Frontispiece showing Fernel seated with a book behind a table at which are the two Heurnes, with patients, a woman and a man, the latter's pulse being felt. Background the interior of a hospital. The order of the works is as in no. 85 (except that the 'Dialogue' follows the Consilia). To the

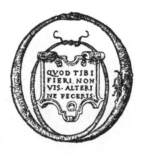

LVGDVNI,
Apud Ioan. Tornæfium, & Gulielmum Gazeium.
1 5 4 8.

Fig. 26.

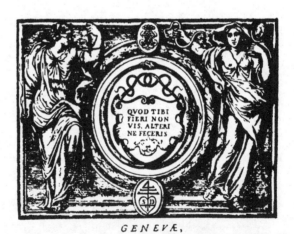

GENEVÆ,

Fig. 27.

Figs. 26, 27. Emblem of the de Tournes' press at Lyons 1548,
and at Geneva 1680.

'Life' a marginal is added giving 1485 as the date of birth and the marginal giving the alternative age of fifty-two is omitted. Among the appreciations following the 'Life' that of the historian de Thou is printed as giving Fernel's age at death as seventy-two. Goulin points out that Guy Patin complained of this as a mistake and asserted it should be fifty-two. The 'Dialogue' is separately paragraphed for the speakers. Misprints are rather plentiful. Goulin complains of the unnecessary inversion of the original order of Fernel's works. About thirty 'cases' by the Heurnes are intercalated. Contains letters between Peter van Bruhesen (q.v.), of Bruges, and Jac. Sylvius, and Fernel, on the illness of Louis of Flanders. A consilium by Fernel is for Louis' consort Eleanor of Austria. The *De Luis Venereae* etc. has marginals. Dr Sinclair finds in this edition a number of typographical variants.

87.J31. Samuel de Tournes, Geneva, 1679. 2°. Pp. 32+814 (misprinted 914)+34. SG, UG. Edited by Théophile Bonet, physician to Henry of Orleans, Duc de Longueville. Th. Bonet (1620–89), of Geneva, of french extraction, practised at Geneva, and then took charge of Henry of Orleans who was deaf from childhood. Bonet gave himself to morbid anatomy. He died of hydrophobia. Contains Plancy's 'Life' of Fernel; also the commentary and cases by the Heurnes. A medallion copper-plate portrait of Fernel by P. Pinchard; Goulin says unrecognizable as a likeness; it seems modelled on the medallion woodcut portrait in V. Andreas' *Imagines Doctorum Vivorum e variis Gentibus*, Antwerp, D. Martinus, 1611. Below it, a Latin couplet by Charles Spon, Dean of Faculty at Lyons, the correspondent and friend of Guy Patin, and editor of Cardan's *Opera Omnia*. 2°. 10 vols. Lugduni, 1663; Title in black and red, and has the device of de Tournes in a medallion supported by two robed figures. Figs. 26 and 27. Index still contains 'that the anima is the cause of the acts of the body and is in man immortal'.

The de Tournes' press had left Lyons for Geneva after St Bartholomew's, but the device and motto are like those on the Lyons issues of 1548 [*v.s.* 6.D3] and 1551 [9.E2], i.e. two snakes forming a circle round a cartouche carrying in four lines *Quod tibi | fieri non | vis, alteri | ne feceris ||*. The title says '*auctior adjectione Encheiridii medico-practici, incerti authoris, et chirurgici Chalmetei*, i.e. of Antoine Chaumette, author of *Enchiridion chirurgicum*, a favourite handbook of surgery, first issued in Paris, 1560, 8°. Brit. Museum has six successive editions.

Title reads:

Johannis | Fernelii | Ambiani | Galliarum Archiatris | Universa Medicina, | Primum Studio & diligentiâ Gulielmi Plantii Cenomani elimata, | Postea | Notis, Observationibus et Remediis Secretis, | Johann. & Othonis Heurni, Ultraject. & aliorum praestantissimorum medicorum Scholiis illustrata, cum | casibus, et observationibus rarioribus, | Ex diario Practico

Othonis Heurni, in Academia Leydensi Primarii | Med. Practicae, Anatomiae & Chirurgiae Professoris annotatis.

Nunc demum operâ Theophili Boneti, Serenissimi quondam Principis Henrici Aureliani, Longa Villae Ducis etc Medici, auctior adjectione Encheiridii Medico-practice incerti Authoris, & Chirurgici Chalmetei, adeò ut singula illorum capita singulis Pathologiae Fernelii capitis (sic) respondunt. Duplici cum Indice, altero capitum, altero Rerum & Verborum locupletissimo.

The 'Dialogue' is paragraphed per speaker. Portrait said to be at age of 52.

88.J32.   Samuel de Tournes, Geneva, 1680.   2°.   Bd, RSM (Clifford Allbutt's copy, 36 cm.; brass clasps), SG, HMS². A reissue of no. 87 including misprints. The last issue of the 'Universal Medicine'.

K.   *Therapeutices universalis* (apart from *Universa Medicina*)   1571

89.K1.   Sebastian Honorat, Lyons, 1571.   8°.   MFP, HMS.   d. 1572.

90.K2.   Louis Cloquemin and Stephan Michel, Lyons, 1574.   8° (small).   BN, CUL, F, TrC, HMS, CSS. Cloquemin also of Geneva, huguenot; Michel extreme huguenot, working with Cloquemin 1573–81.

91.K3.   Les sept livres de la Thérapeutique Universelle de M. Jean Fernel, traduit par le Sieur Du Teil. Jean Guignard père et fils, Paris, 1648.   8°.   BN, MFP.

92.K4.   As no. 91 but 1655.   MFP, F, CSS.

93.K5.   As no. 91 but 1668.   BN, Vat.   Claims to be a fresh translation, but is in fact that of Du Teil almost word for word (Goulin).

L.   *Touching the outward Affects of the Body*, trans. by W. Clowes
1575

94.L.   (*Seventh book of the 'Pathology', i.e. Surgical; in English*, 1575.) A new and approved treatise concerning the cure of the French Pockes by the unctions, whereunto is adjoined a right learned work touching the outward affects of the body, written by the learned physician and chirurgeon Fernelius, etc. by William Clowes, Chirurgeon of London. *London*, 1575. 8°. Copies: I have found no copy. Mentioned by Astruc. (vol. II, bk 6: *De Morbis Venereis*), who accepts it as being the bk. 7 'On External Diseases', of the 'Pathology'. The short-title catalogue of English books to 1640 does not mention it. Goulin points out that the views on surgery attributed by Haller to Fernel on the basis of this book are a mistake of Haller's. The author is Wm. Clowes the Elder, who became surgeon to Queen Elizabeth (Sir Wm. Clowes). He was well acquainted with french and latin. The book had successive reissues up to 1637. There is a 'Briefe & necessarie Treatise' on *lues venerea* by Clowes, London, 1585.

M. *Febrium Curandarum Methodus Generalis* 1577

95.M1. Febrium curandarum methodus generalis. Andreas Wechel, Frankfort, 1577. 8°. Prelim. + 94 pp. AU, BN. Editor, Jean Lamy, M.D., of Paris; dedicated from Paris, September 1577, to Jean Barjotte, Seigneur of Marcheffrai, grandson of Jean Fernel and eldest son of Philibert, Knight and President of the Pretorian Council. A long letter stating that Fernel during his lifetime was exposed to bitter jealousy. It mentions the two works found complete by Plancy at Fernel's death, this on Fevers being one, and that on *lues venerea* the other. It says that Plancy's death has frustrated the intention to publish them, and Lamy now undertakes it. He has taken counsel with Barjotte about it. The memory of Fernel is being injured by garbled versions of the work; *victis nil nisi dolor.*

96.M2. Heirs of A. Baldo, Rome, 1579. 8°. F. The tract was included in the Wechel folio volume of 1577 containing the *Universa Medicina* and in vol. III of the 8° of 1581, and in many subsequent editions, e.g. the 1592 folio. In the folio of 1578 the letter from Lamy was not included, but it is given in the 1581 4° and in the 1592 folio and a number of subsequent editions. It was not again published separately, except as item no. 97, in french in the seventeenth century.

97.M3. Translation into french by Charles de Saint German, physician to the king; privilege to the relict of Jean le Bouc, April 1638, who transferred it to Guignard, father and son. Paris, 1655. 12°. HMS.

N. *De Luis Venereae perfectissima Cura Liber* 1579

98.N1. De luis Venereae curatione perfectissima liber. Plantin, Antwerp, 1579. 8°. BM, Bd, SG, UG. Dedicatory letter from Victor Giselinus to Jean Douza à Noortwijck. Plantin printed from a MS. obtained by Giselinus from Fr. Rapaert of Bruges. Goulin thinks J. Lamy had also a MS. in 1571. See Goulin, *Mém.* p. 367.

Of Jean Douza (Van der Does) 'dominus à Noortwijck' two engraved portraits exist, one in his *Nova Poemata*, 8°, Leiden, 1575, and another in part 4 of J. J. Boissard's *Icones Virorum Illustrium Doctrina et Eruditione Praestantium ad Vivum Effictae*, 4°, Frankfort, 1599. Both are full-page engravings, the latter by T. de Bry. Following the text is a 12-page letter, dated Bruges, August 1579, by Giselinus to Martin Everart, 'Opinions of some other learned men on the use of Mercury'. Goulin says he has not found this in the three copies of the volume accessible to him. Astruc mentions the letter. The British Museum copy has it; the University of Glasgow copy not. It was included as pp. 60–63 in the copy of no. 65 seen by Goulin, who suggested that it had been included in some only of the copies, and had '1580' printed on it, not forestalling Plantin's issue of 1579. Does was at the College de Coqueret with Dorat.

99.N2. Paul Mejetti, Padua, 1580. 8°. Goulin had not seen a copy, and I have not been able to trace one.
The *De Luis Venereae Curatione* subsequently appeared in various collections of Fernel. Thus, in the *Universa Medicina* of 1581 (Wechel) and again in the *Universa Medicina*, 1592 (Wechel), and in nos. 81, 85, 86, 87. It appeared in the *Aphrodiseas*, Christian Henry Cuno's heirs, Jena, 1789, 2°, by C. G. Grüner, containing writings missed by the *Aphrodisiacus* of Luvigini. Grüner contributed a notice of Fernel to the *Almanach der Aerzte*, 1789, p. 180: BM, CSS, etc. It was also in the 'Collection' of writers on 'Morbus Gallicus', by Grüner, issued by the University Press, Jena, 1793, 8°: RPEd. In this collection it is copied from the Wechel issue of 1592; Grüner was seemingly unaware of Wechel's earlier issue of it.

100.N3. Nicolas de la Coste, Paris, 1633. 12°. BN. In french by Michel le Long, DM. Le Pileur remarks on the badness of this translation. Goulin on the badness of the paper. Michel le Long translated also and annotated a *Schola Salernitana* issued in 18° in 1633, and is described as 'Provinois' This *Schola Salernitana* ran into four editions by 1649.

101.N4. Masson et Cie, Paris, 1879. 8°. French and latin, trans. with notes by L. le Pileur. BM, BN, F, CSS, etc. Le Pileur took as text that of 1581 included in no. 68 *supra*. Le Pileur dismisses Le Long's translation as 'laisse fort à désirer'.

P.   *La Chirurgie*   1579

102.P1. (In french.) Le Chirurgie de Fernel, translatée de latin illustrée de briefues annotations et d'une methode chirurgique, par Simon Provanchières, médecin à Sens, et de Monseigneur...Cardinal de Guise and Duc de Rheims, premier pair de France. Imprimé par J. Savine, Sens, 1579. 12°. Goulin saw this and found it a commentary as much as a translation of the seventh book of the *Pathologia*. On sale in Paris by G. Chaudière, rue St Jacques at the sign 'du Temps et de l'homme sauvage'. I have found no copy.

103.P2. J. Bosc, Toulouse, 1666. 12°. HMS.

104.P3. As no. 103 but 1667. 12°.

Q.   *Consilium pro epileptico*   1580

105.Q1. Consilium pro epileptico scriptum. Andrew Wechel, Frankfort, 1580. 8°. BN. This is one of four short tracts contained in a volume entitled *Medicamentorum facile parabilium adversus omnis generis articulorum dolores enumeratio ab Antonio Schneebergero*, of Zurich, M.D. Fernel's *Consilium* is prefaced by Sneeberger, '13 Nov 1579 from my house in

Cracow'. This is its first publication. It was not in the *Liber Consiliorum* issued by Capel in 1582 nor in Capel's re-issues. But it was included in the collected editions of Fernel published in 1597, 1602, 1605, 1607, 1610, 1619, and in the Leyden edition of 1645, where it heads the other Consilia. In a copy of the 1607 *Universa Medicina* Goulin found it bearing many corrections and some additions in MS., taken from a MS. copy belonging to Dalechamps, the contemporary of Laurent Joubert from Lyons. Two MSS. of this Consilium so widely apart as Cracow and Montpellier were thus in existence after Fernel's death, although Capel in Paris had no copy along with the other Fernel Consilia. Anton S. died in Cracow, 1581.

106.Q2.   B. Albin. Speyer, 1592. 8°. F.

R.   *Consiliorum Medicinalium Liber* 1582

107.R1.   Consiliorum Medicinalium Liber. Ægidius Beys, Paris, 1582. 8°. Pp. 144. Vat, BN, F, CSS. Has a dedicatory letter from Gulielmus Capellus, D.M. Paris, to D. Juan de Paulmier. Le Paulmier was a pupil of Fernel, as was Capell. Le Paulmier was excluded from the Faculty in 1564, with others, for being of the 'reformed faith' (Wickersheimer, p. 38). He controverted Paré on the treatment of gunshot wounds. Capell states that these Consilia, seventy-nine in number, are selected from four hundred Consilia from the notebooks of his teacher, Fernel. Gilles Beyes was a son-in-law of Christophe Plantin, and started printing in Antwerp; in Paris, 1577, rue St Jacques, 'au lys blanc'.

108.R2.   John Wechel, Frankfort, 1584. 8°. RPEd, SG.

109.R3.   Ægidius Beys, Paris, 1585. 8°. BN, CSS. The letter by Capell is expanded, with further information about Fernel. Part of it runs: 'Twenty years ago I was attracted by the honeyed eloquence and pithy judgments of this great man. In his crucible everything was reduced to certainty. Greek, latin, or whatever else, he took their living threads and wove them into a texture at once rich and apposite. He had the gift of choosing and combining into a just whole'. 'Hence, when I had lectured publicly on his "Physiology", I wanted to re-issue his consultations and remedies, and sought out yourself, and re-kindled the interest of our publishers in this compendium, so that it might see the light, with your good help. And that has now come to pass in its issue both here and, at the same time, in Germany (et à Germanicis semel)'. This refers to the edition from Frankfort in the same year, 1585, by A. Wechel, Fernel's Paris publisher, who, in 1574, had moved to Frankfort.

   The 'index' contains references to 125 ff. but the book stops with *finis* on f. 112. An item in the index runs '*contra mulierculas medicinam factitantes*', f. 125; I find in the book nothing answering to this. Nor has the index of the 1582 edition anything corresponding with it. The Epilogue in de Bethencourt's 'Carême', summing up 'Mercury', says: 'Qu'on l'accuse d'insuccès nombreux, cela n'a rien qui doive nous surprendre, car nous le voyons journellement prescrit sans règle ni raison par des charlatans, des empiriques, des imposteurs de tout genre, voire même par des courtisanes.' A. Fournier's transl. Paris, 1871, p. 93.

110.R4. John Wechel, Frankfort, 1585. 8°. Pp. 144. BN, F, HMS, CSS.
The letter by Capell is that of 1582 unaltered.

111.R5. Gio. Dominic Tarino, Turin, 1589. 8°. Vat, CSS. Dedicated to Jerome Ardizonius, chief physician to Queen Christina of Denmark, Norway, Sweden, etc. Countess of Bablon and Tortona.

112.R6. John Wechel, Frankfort, 1593. 8°. BM, AU², BN, Bd, RS, SG, UG.

113.R7. Peter de la Rovière, Orleans, 1604. 8°. F, HMS.

114.R8. Heirs of Marny, Hanau, 1610. 8°. CUL², TrC².

115.R9. Franc. Hacke, Leyden, 1644. 8°. AU, CUL, CSL, GCC, RSM, SG, HSM, TrC.

116.R10. (In english.) Select Medicinal Counsels of J. Fernel. J. Streeter, sold by G. Sawbridge, Ludgate Hill, London. 1657. 2°. Translated by N. Culpepper, Abdiah Cole and William Rowland (with four books of L. Riverius). MSL, HC.

117.R11. As no. 116, 1658. CUL, EU, MLM.

118.R12. As no. 116, 1670. MSL.

119.R13. As no. 116, 1672. BM, AU.

120.R14. As no. 116, 1678. CSL, MLM.

121.R15. As no. 116, 1688. RSM.

S.   *De Morbo Articulari*   1592

122.S. De morbo articulari. In 'de arthritidis praeservatione and curatione consilia, opera H. Garetii edita'. John Wechel and Peter Fischer, partners, Frankfort, 1592. 8°. AU. Contains a Consilium on arthritis sent to Pierre Bruhesius, physician to Eleanor of Austria, second wife of Francis I of France. Goulin thinks the letter was written early in 1548, because it promises to send next winter a copy of the 'dialogus de abditis rerum causis', when this latter will have appeared in print.

T. *Medici Antiqui* 1594

123.T. Medici antiqui; graeci, latini, atque arabes, qui de febribus scripserunt, in unum collecti ab excell. D. Joanne Fernelio, ambiano. Robert Mejetti, Venice, 1594. 2°. CSL, RPEd. (? Any connection with Fernel except the insertion of his name on the title-page.)

U. *Pharmacia* 1605

124.U, Pharmacia | Jo. Fernelii | *cum* | Guiliel | Planti | et | Franc, Saguyeri | Scholiis: | *in usum* | pharmacopoeorum | nunc primum edita. | Hanoviae | *typis Wechelianis*, apud | *Claud. Marnium et haeredes Jo. Aubrii.* | (Hanau), 1605. Dedication and preface 10 pp. + 348 pp. + 8 pp. index. 12°. BN, MFP, AU, GCC, MSL. Dedicatory letter from Caspar Bauhin, Professor of Anatomy and Botany, University of Basle, dated 16 December, 1604.

This is an edition of bk. vii ('On Prescriptions') of the 'Therapeutics' of the 'Universal Medicine', with, additional to the notes of Plancy, notes by Francis Saguyer, M.D. Bauhin inscribes it to a youthful patron, a Moravian, of noble birth, whose parents also come in for mention in the dedicatory letter. The letter gives as reason for the publication that though each country has its recognized prescriptions, and in Italy almost every city—Rome, Florence, Bologna, Ferrara, Mantua, Bergamo—the prescriptions of Fernel are so especially elegant that they are in favour far outside France itself. Bauhin republishes them that they may be better obtainable, and as a mark of respect to the old physician Saguyer of Bourgogne, and further to oblige the 'learned and able' apothecary, Jean Legros of Langres, who has sent to him the commentary on them by Saguyer, as yet unpublished and additional to the commentary by Guillaume Plancy in the 'Universal Medicine'. Bauhin speaks of Plancy as 'nephew of Fernel'. Goulin (1775), in a footnote, p. 323, says that M. Andry, a regent of the Paris Faculty, engaged in writing the history of the Faculty, tells him that Plancy married a niece of Fernel and had a son who became a priest and died in 1638, and that Andry gave the date of Plancy's death as 1568.

Bauhin's letter is succeeded by a Preface from Francis Saguyer. This is addressed to all practitioners of Hippocratic and Galenical medicine; it rebukes spagyrical treatment which 'a certain flock follow'. Saguyer mentions having listened to Fernel and Sylvius in Paris, and been a pupil of Rondelet in Montpellier. He extols Fernel and says his 'Physiology' and 'Pathology' are recognized everywhere as beyond praise. Saguyer's commentaries give long notes on many of the prescriptions, e.g. on 'theriac' and 'Mithridate', which he says have a similar action. He discusses Fernel's receipts for these. He denies that Mithridates, King of

Pontus, was inventor of the antidote bearing his name; he says it was 'the physicians Antipater and Cleophantes'. Goulin has interesting remarks on Saguyer, and regrets his commentary was never republished.

W.   Two Treatises on Eyesight   1616

125.W1. Two treatises concerning the preservation of eyesight, and out of those famous physicians Fernelius and Riolanus, the first written by Dr J. Baily, sometime of Oxford. Joseph Barnes for John Barnes, Oxford, 1616. 8°. BM, Bd, RSM. Baily was a physician to Queen Elizabeth, was educated at Winchester and Oxford, and took his M.D. in 1563. He became Regius Professor at Oxford.

126.W2. Directions for health, etc. with two treatises on Diseases of the eyes, by Dr Baily and by Fernelius, by Sir W. Vaughan. John Beale for Francis Williams, London, 1626. 4°. BM, Bd, CUL, RSM.

127.W3. Another edition. By Thomas Harper for John Harison, London, 1633. 4°. Bd, MLM, MSL. An enlarged edition of no. 126.

X.   Pathologia (by itself)   1638

128.X1. Pathologia, libri septem, Jean de Mire, Paris, 1638. 12°. BN, MFP. Describes itself as 'new edition', fully corrected. Prefaced by a letter (November 1637) from two publishers, Cl. Groult and J. de Mire, to Guy Patin, Dean of the Faculty. Goulin suggests that the notices of Fernel in this letter were written by Patin himself. The verso of p. 8 has a new engraved portrait of Fernel in an oval. Under it the year of his birth is given as 1506, and that he 'denatus' 1558, at the age of fifty-two. Goulin shows that this date of birth was in agreement with a view strongly held by Patin. Indeed, it would seem that Patin, when dean and in charge of the records of the Faculty, eighty years or so after Fernel's death, inserted that age—not originally mentioned—in the records. The right age, Goulin establishes, was sixty-two. Contains the latin elegiacs on Fernel signed N. Borbonius, thought by Goulin to be written at request of Patin.

129.X2. (In french.) La Pathologie de Jean Fernel, premier medecin de Henry II, Roy de France, Ouvrage tres-utile a tous ceux qui s'appliquent a la connoissance du Corps humain. Mis en Francois, par A.D.M. Docteur en Medecine. A Paris, chez Jean Guignard, au premier pilier de la grand-salle du Palais, proche les consultations. 1650. Issued for the surgeons who were not taught latin. Privilege du Roy, 29 Avril 1638 to Widow Jean le Bouc, for Les Œuvres de Jean Fernel all or in part for nine years to count from the day on which the printing is finished; 'achevé d'imprimer 23 Avril 1646'. 8°. F, CSS. This translation was from the Pathologia of the Medicina (1554), not from that of the Universa Medicina

(1567); it omits the 'appendicitis' case (bk. vi, c. 9). The 'surgeons' of St Côme and the 'barber-surgeons' united in 1646.

130.X3. As no. 129, 1655. BN, MFP

131.X4. As no. 129, 1660. F.

132.X5. As no. 129, 1665. HMS.

133.X6. The *Pathologia* from the Bonet edition; *v.s.* 87.J31; Geneva, 1683. 12°. RSM.

Y. *De Morbis Universalibus et Particularibus* 1645

134.Y. The last four books of the *Pathologia*. Fr. Hackius, Leyden, 1645. 8°. HMS, RSM. With engraving on title of Fernel standing, in cap and gown, addressing a man, seated, with a crutch; same as in no. 85. Uniform with nos. 115 and 85.

Z. *De Febribus, pathologiae Liber quartus* 1664

135.Z. Joannis Fernelii pathologiae liber quartus de febribus. Ægidius Valkenier, Amstelodam. MDLXIV (misprint for 1664). 8° (small). MSL, MFP, HMS, with a commentary by Rutger Loenius, physician and professor of philosophy, of Amsterdam. With a lengthy eulogy of Fernel and his work.

GHOSTS

De Naturali Parte Medicinae. Paris, 1545, 8°, Venice, 1545, 8°.

De abditis rerum causis. Paris, 1552, 2°. Asserted by Theo. Georgius, *Bücher Lexikon*, Leipsic, 1742 and by P. G. Boisseau, *Biographie Médicale*, Paris, 1821, vol. IV. Goulin questioned the existence of this edition (p. 359).

Universa Medicina. Francfort, Marny and Aubry, 1603, 8°. Given by Kerstner.

Therapeutices universalis seu medendi rationis lib. VII. Paris, 1554, 8°.

Therapeutices universalis seu medendi rationis lib. Lyon, 1564, 8°.

Georgi. Goulin (p. 378) questions this. Utrecht, 1686, questioned by Goulin (p. 379).

Febrium curandarum methodus generalis. Paris, 1554, 2°; Venice, 1555, 8°; Venice, 1564, 4°; Paris, 1567, 2°.

Pathologia. Frankfort, 1592, 2°.

Chronology of Events

1493 Columbus returns from discovery of America.

1497 Fernel's birth (Goulin).

1508 Guiac wood first brought from America.

1509 Henry VIII king of England.

1511 Erasmus at Cambridge.

1515 Accession of Francis I.

1516 Fernel enters Ste Barbe, University of Paris. More's *Utopia*.

1518 Linacre (Wolsey) founds the College of Physicians, London. 'Bibliothèque Royale' started in France.

1519 Fernel's M.A. degree. Charles elected Emperor.

1521 Berengario doubts if the heart's septum lets through blood or spirit (Galen).

1522 Magellan completes the voyage round the world. Rhodes taken by Solyman.

1524 Fernel enters on University course for M.D. Linacre founds lectures on Medicine at Oxford and Cambridge.

1525 Battle of Pavia.

1526 Fernel resident in Ste Barbe and lecturing on philosophy (Aristotle).

1527 Fernel's *Monalosphaerium* published. The German sack and pillage of Rome.

1528 Fernel's *Cosmotheoria* published (March). Fernel's *De Proportionibus* published (November).

1530 Francis I founds Chairs of Greek and Hebrew at Paris.

1530 Fernel's M.D. degree. Death of Wolsey.

1531–2 Fernel settles in Paris, and marries.

1535 Rabelais' *Gargantua*. Jesuit order founded.

1535 Fernel relinquishes 'mathematics'.

1536 Fernel teaching medicine in Collège de Cornouailles; begins writing *De naturali parte Medicinae*.

1540 Death of Budé. Barber-Surgeons incorporated in London.

1542 Fernel's *De naturali parte Medicinae* published; the 'Dialogue' has been written and circulated in MS. Appointed a physician to the dauphin. Étienne Dolet's *Cicero's Letters*, at Lyons.

1543 Copernicus' *De Revolutionibus* published.

1544 Catherine de Medicis' first child born, Fernel her physician. St Bartholomew's Hospital, London, refounded (under Thomas Vicary).

1545 Fernel's *De Vacuandi Ratione* published. Fernel summoned to Diane de Poitiers; she recovers.

1546 Étienne Dolet burned in Paris.

1547 Henri II succeeds Francis I. Fernel's younger daughter born. Henry VIII died.

1548 Fernel's *De Abditis Rerum Causis* (the 'Dialogues') published. Regius Professorship of Physic founded at Cambridge.

1550 Fernel's practice too large to allow him to lecture.

1551 P. Ramus appointed professor (Paris) by Henri II.

1553 Mary succeeds Edward VI of England. Servetus burned as a heretic, Geneva.

1554 Fernel's *Medicina* published.

1555 At work on completing the 'Therapeutics': is a physician-in-ordinary to the king.

1556–7 Appointed physician-in-chief to the king: the *De Luis Venereae Curatione* being written; also further 'Therapeutics'. Is accompanying the king in the campaign.

1558 Calais taken by Duke of Guise. Fernel returns to the Court (Fontainebleau): his wife dies of fever. He then develops fever and dies, 26 April.

1567 A. Wechel publishes the *Universa Medicina*, editor G. Plancy.

1568 ? Death of Plancy.

Index

common sensorium, 81, 84
Community of the Master Barber-surgeons, 112
concepts, 79
conjunctions of the planets, 29, 30, 36, 186
consilia, 38, 101
Consiliorum Medicinalium Liber, 58, 126, 203
Consilium pro Epileptico, 202, 203
Constantinople, 179
Constantinus, Balthazar (Venice), 195
contagion (rabies), 131, 132
contraries, 43, 117
control of movement, 88; reflex, 88
Cook, James, of Warwick, 75
Copernicus, Nicolas (1473–1543), 67, 208
Copland, W., 24
Cordier, Mathurin, 12, 14
Cornarius, Janus (Johan Hagenbut) (1500–58), 66
Cosmotheoria, 15, 173, 188
Costa ben Luca, 84
Coste, Nicolas de la (Paris), 202
cowpox, 124
Cracow, 203
Crato, Johannes (of Kraftheim) (1519–85), 137, 148
'critical days', 33, 98, 159
Crooke, 92
Crump, Lucy, 62
Culpepper, N., 204
cures, magical, 42
Cushing, Harvey, 95

Dale, Sir Henry, 97, 119
Daleschamps, Jacques (of Lyons) (1530–88), 109
Dampier, Sir William, 51
Dauphiné, 108, 203
Dean, Professor H. R., 184
Deas, Mr Henry, 60
death, 39; Descartes on, 83; Fernel on, 80
decrees against quackery, 23
Denny-Brown, Professor D., ix
Descartes, 79, 81, 84, 86, 88, 139
Destrebey, Jacques-Louis, 15, 16
Deventer, 8

dialectics, 2, 3
Dialogues, 16, 35, 40, 52, 53, 191, 192; commentaries on, 22; date of, 22, 174
Diane de Poitiers, 10, 53, 63, 156, 190, 198, 209
diastole, 74
Diderot, Denis (1713–83), 24
dissection, 64
Dissectione, De, 64
Doctrinale, 7
Dôle, 120
Dolet, Étienne, 34, 208, 209
Donation of Constantine, 124
Dorat, 201
Douza, Jean (Jan van der Does), 201
Dupuys, Jacques (Paris), 192
Dusseau, Michel, 105
Du Teil, 200

Eberhard of Béthune, 8
Écoles de Santé, 56
Edinburgh, Coll. of Physicians' Library, 187; University Library, 187
editions of Fernel, list of, 187–207
Edward III, 48
Egypt, 128
'egyptian days', 98
Eleanor of Austria, 121, 204
elemental heat, 38
elements, 64, 65
elixir, 48, 50
Elizabeth of England, 104, 130, 179, 200
Empedocles, 64
empirics, 111
Encyclopèdie, 24
endocarditis, 102
England, war with, 163
ephemerides, 27
epilepsy, 36, 37
Erasmus, Desiderius (1466–1536), 6, 8, 11, 52, 123, 184, 208
Erastus, Thomas (1525–83), 31, 33, 45, 52
Erreurs Populaires, 90, 107, 114, 185
Estienne, Charles ((Paris) son of 'Henri I'), 9
Estienne, Henri, 9, 112 (Paris)
Estienne, Henri (Paris, then Geneva), son of Robert, 111, 180

Compass: W · S · N · E

Pte St. Michel · R. de la Harpe · St. Côme · St. Dami

Coll. d. Cluny

R. de la K Sorbonne · R. d. Mathurins

les Jacobins · Coll. de Calvi G · Sorbonne · St. Benoit · P N

R. S a i n t · J a c q u e s

Pte. St. Jacques · St. Etienne de Grés

Coll. des Langres · Coll. du Plessis · H r. Fromentel · Coll de Cambrai · F ED · Coll. Treguier · Cr. St. J. La tran

r. Cholets · R. St. Jean de · Cr R B

Coll. Mont-aigu S · Coll. de S. Barbe · C. de Rheims · Coll. Coqueret · Beauvais · Canon Law Sch. · Coll. de Beauv

Coll. de Lisieux

Coll. de Fortet · Coll. M des Italiens · Coll. Laon

Ste Geneviève · R. de Mont St. Genevi

r. de Bordelle · Coll. de Navarre

A · Coll. de Tournai

A. S. de Colines, 4 Evangelistes,1539; B. S. de Colines, Soleil d'Or; 15
C. Pegasus (formerly Jeu-de-Paume), C, Wechel (formerly Perier) 15
D. Ecu-de-Basle Chr. Wechel. E. Compas-d'Or, A. Perier (Plantin) Gilles B

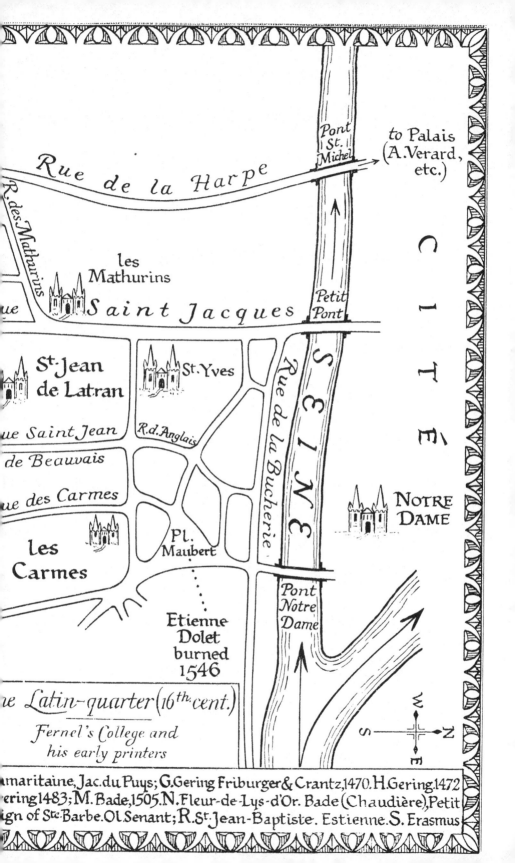

Rue de la Harpe

R. des Mathurins

R. des Mathurins

Rue

les Mathurins

Saint Jacques

St·Jean de Latran

St. Yves

Rue Saint Jean de Beauvais

R. d. Anglais

Rue des Carmes

Rue de la Bucherie

les Carmes

Pl. Maubert

Etienne Dolet burned 1546

Pont St. Michel

to Palais (A. Verard, etc.)

Petit Pont

SEINE

CITE

NOTRE DAME

Pont Notre Dame

W · N · E · S

The Latin-quarter (16th. cent.)

Fernel's College and his early printers

...maritaine, Jac. du Puys; G. Gering Friburger & Crantz, 1470. H. Gering 1472
...ering 1483; M. Bade, 1505. N. Fleur-de-Lys-d'Or. Bade (Chaudière), Petit
...ign of Ste. Barbe. Ol. Senant; R. St. Jean-Baptiste. Estienne. S. Erasmus

Printed in the United States
By Bookmasters